THE DIABETES DIET:

*How To Manage Your Diet For Weight Loss
And Incredible Blood Sugar Control*

2ND Edition

**Dr Katharine Morrison
and Emma Baird**

Published by Pink Glitter Publishing

ISBN: 978-1-9997738-1-6

Cover design and interior layout: Bogdan Matei

CONTENTS

DISCLAIMER

This book is copyrighted with all rights reserved. The authors cannot assume any liability for the misuse of information contained within this book. The authors intend the information provided in this book to be used as advice which can help to improve your health and well-being. It is important to note, however, that the book has been co-written by an author who is not a healthcare professional and neither does she claim to be.

Please consult your doctor and your healthcare team before setting out on any programme of nutrition, exercise, or remedy. By consulting your primary care physician, you will be better placed to understand and address your particular symptoms and situation in the most effective way possible. Following a low-carbohydrate diet may result in lower blood sugar levels, and if you are taking any blood sugar lowering medication, this must be taken into account. Low-blood sugar levels must be treated as soon as possible with fast-acting carbohydrates, even if you are following a low-carbohydrate diet.

While every attempt has been made to provide information that is accurate and useful, the authors cannot make any guarantees that the remedies presented within this book will help everyone in every situation. Individual histories, physical conditioning, body type, underlying conditions all play a part in a person's history, so results will vary.

INTRODUCTION TO
THE 2ND EDITION

Since we wrote The Diabetes Diet for weight loss and incredible blood sugar control in 2014, there has been increasing acceptance that a low carb diet is not just the most effective diet for diabetes management, but it is the best for cardiovascular disease prevention as well. There have also been effects on the reduction of cancer and degenerative diseases.

There are now many low carb books out there, and you may be wondering what this book especially has to offer. Our book is particularly relevant to people who have type one diabetes and people with type two diabetes who use insulin because we give highly detailed help with insulin management and the transition to a low carb diet. Few books grapple with this because of the complex nature of the changes that need to be made for optimal blood sugar control.

At the same time, we look after those people who are on medications for their type two diabetes, those with pre-diabetes, polycystic ovarian syndrome and those who just wish to lose some body fat. We help women planning a pregnancy, children, young adults, adults of working age and older adults.

We know that blood sugar targets need to be set for the individual and that everyone will have different requirements regarding optimal total carbohydrate intake. We, therefore, explore the range of ways of practising low carbohydrate dietary techniques including those who prefer a meat-free eating plan.

The American Association of Clinical Endocrinologists in the USA and the Royal College of General Practitioners in the UK, are promoting low carbohydrate diets for diabetics now and we hope that as demand for information grows this book will fill an unmet need not only for patients and carers but for medical professionals. We are particularly pleased to bring out our new edition in print as well as in e-book format.

Dr Katharine Morrison and Emma Baird, October 17. Visit our blog at: https://diabetesdietblog.com

INTRODUCTIONS

Hello and welcome to The Diabetes Diet. How are you feeling right now?

We ask this question as it is more than likely you have picked up this book for one of two reasons – either you want to lose weight, or you are attracted by the idea of incredible blood sugar control. The two often go hand in hand, as blood sugars which remain stable throughout the day and the night result in less hunger, which in turn leads to a naturally regulated appetite and that means you are more likely to lose weight.

Are you fed up with your diabetes? Tired of getting variable blood sugar levels, which seem to happen no matter how strictly you follow that prescribed low-fat diet with its recommendations of plenty of "healthy" foods such as wholemeal bread and pasta, brown rice and beans?

Or are you just tired in general? Do you feel as if you need a nap after every meal and do you long for weekends when you don't need to get up quite so early for work?

Do you get days when even the thought of talking to your fellow human beings seems exhausting, and do your family, friends and work colleagues tip-toe around you a lot of the time, afraid that you will lash out? Grumpiness and depression often accompany tiredness after all... That is, of course, if you have any energy left to lash out.

For the majority of those with diabetes, diabetic complications can seem inevitable.

Yet, complications can be minimised, reduced completely, or even reversed by good enough blood sugar management. The biggest problem has been the failure to teach people to eat the right foods that make blood sugar management easy[1].

Next is the inability to match insulin well enough to these foods. These topics are not taught with the thoroughness they deserve at most diabetic clinics. This book aims to redress this issue.

Let me introduce myself and this book's co-author – my name is Emma Baird, and I have type 1 diabetes, diagnosed when I was aged 9 in 1982. I started exploring low-carbohydrate diets four years ago, and I have followed such diets ever since as I believe they hold the secret to better health and better energy levels.

… And I am Dr Katharine Morrison. I am a general practitioner, with a busy practice in Ayrshire, Scotland. My son was diagnosed with type 1 diabetes in 2004, which led me to investigate ways in which I could improve his health, minimise his chances of suffering low blood sugar episodes and improve his long-term blood sugar results also known as the HbA1C.

My son has achieved average HbA1 results of 6.5 % over the last 10 years. The range has been 4.8-7.2% with a current level of 5.8%. This is all the more remarkable when you consider that he became diabetic on the cusp of puberty which is a notoriously difficult time to achieve reasonable blood sugars. The average HbA1c for 16-25-year-olds in the UK is about 10.1%, and there has been no improvement to this in decades, despite the variety of insulins and devices now available.[2]

Good HbA1c results are significant if a person with diabetes is to reduce their risk of developing diabetes-related complications, such as the increased risk of heart disease, strokes, non-traumatic amputations, kidney failure and blindness.

I have worked extensively with patients who have both type 1 and type 2 diabetes at my practice and online, encouraging them to follow a low-carbohydrate diet and manage their medications accordingly. Every patient who has diligently followed a low carbohydrate diet has achieved lowered HbA1 results and improvements in their energy levels, as well as losing weight if this was something that they needed to do.

We wrote this book together for anyone with type 1 or 2 diabetes who wants to know how to manage their blood sugars or weight with a low-carbohydrate diet.

Those with a professional interest in low-carbohydrate diets can learn from this book and thus offer a safe and effective way to lose body fat, keep it off, and obtain normal or near normal blood sugars for their own patients.

By eating mainly unrefined, minimally processed foods and matching insulin and blood sugar lowering medications more precisely to meals, you can avoid the damaging blood glucose spikes that are known to cause ageing of all the tissues of the body. Vascular changes and adverse blood lipid patterns that cause further damage are addressed with a low carbohydrate diet too.

Blood sugar management is good for everyone – diabetes diagnosis or not, as you will discover from the first chapter of our book. If you do not currently suffer from type 2 diabetes and you want to keep it that way, then this book is for you too. Adopting a low-carbohydrate diet can minimise your chances of developing type 2 diabetes in later life – and that also lessens your chances of developing the diabetes-related complications such as heart disease, high blood pressure, stroke, kidney failure and blindness.

What makes our book different is the detailed advice about managing your medication which will transform the management of your diabetes, minimise the number of hypoglycaemic episodes you will experience and give you stable energy levels all day.

Too tired to speak to anyone? Having a grumpy day or dreading the thought of tomorrow's meeting at work scheduled for after lunch, a time you know from previous experience is usually your lowest energy level point of the day?

Prepare for your energy levels to shoot through the roof.

CHAPTER 1

WHAT IS DIABETES AND WHY IS BLOOD SUGAR CONTROL SO IMPORTANT?

Diabetes. Epidemic. Healthcare costs. Ticking time bomb. Diabetes-related complications. Increased risk of heart disease, stroke, kidney failure, non-traumatic amputations and blindness.

These are all words that you will no doubt have heard in the way that people and media outlets use to talk about diabetes these days. If you have the condition yourself, always hearing about diabetes referred to in such ways can be very unnerving indeed. After all, who wants to live with a disease which has so many risks attached?

Many of you reading this book will have diabetes yourself, but if you are newly-diagnosed or you suspect that you are at risk of developing diabetes in the future, here is a quick explanation of the condition and why it puts you at risk of so many health problems.

Diabetes is a widespread, life-long health condition. It happens when the amount of glucose (sugar) in your body is too high because your body cannot use the sugar properly. This is either because your pancreas does not produce insulin (type 1 diabetes) or it can't produce enough insulin, or that the insulin that is produced does not work properly (type 2 diabetes).

Insulin is a hormone, and its role is to transport sugar in the blood to our cells where it is converted to energy. If the sugar in our blood can't enter our cells, then it can't be used as fuel and it builds up as sugar in the blood and diabetes develops. High amounts of sugar in the blood are highly toxic.

There are more than 3.2 million people in the UK[3] who know they have diabetes (and 25.8 million inhabitants in the US[4]). In the UK, about 10% of those 3.2 million people have type 1 diabetes, and around 90% have type 2 diabetes.

Although hospital clinics and GP surgeries do a lot of work to monitor and treat the complications of diabetes, not enough effort is put into prevention of those complications. Poor control of blood sugars, i.e. sugar levels that run at high levels for extended periods of time, is the primary factor that causes complications such as blindness, kidney failure and amputations because of the toxicity of sugar in the blood.

1. 78% of type 1 diabetics attending clinics have what is considered to be unacceptably high blood sugar levels. This equates to HbA1c levels of more than 58mmols, an average blood sugar level of 9.4mmol/l (normal blood sugar levels are 4-6.00mmol or 72-108mg) or in International Federation of Clinical Chemistry (IFCC) units of [79.2mmol/mol].

2. 38% of the total number of type 1 diabetics attending clinics have inferior blood sugar control with blood sugar levels equating to HbA1 levels of more than 9%, an average blood sugar level of 12.6 mmol/l, or an IFCC number of 113mmol/mol.

The development of diabetes-related complications can seem inevitable if you have the condition, but why do high blood sugar levels make you so much more at risk of health problems?

Earlier, we referred to high blood sugar levels as incredibly toxic, and indeed they can have horrible effects on your internal organs, your limbs, your eyes and your skin – in short, there aren't many parts of your body which will not be adversely affected by high blood sugar levels.

Heart disease or stroke. If you have diabetes, you are more likely to get heart disease or a stroke than someone who doesn't have diabetes. This is partially due to damage to the lining of the blood vessels called endothelium caused by high insulin levels. Also, the lipid pattern tends to favour the small, highly oxidised LDL particles that plug up damaged endothelium causing plaques and the nitric oxide system in the blood vessels becomes damaged by blood sugar spikes initiating vascular constriction.[5] These and other factors lead to unstable plaques in arteries and constricted blood vessels. Heart attacks and thrombotic strokes are caused by the interruption of the free flow of oxygenated blood.

Diabetic kidney disease (diabetic nephropathy) results when the filters of the kidneys (glomeruli) of people with diabetes become damaged. Because of the damage, the kidneys begin to leak abnormal amounts of protein into the urine – a condition called proteinuria. If proteinuria is not controlled, the increased level of protein in your urine can lead to more kidney damage which can, over time, cause your kidneys to fail which will require either regular dialysis or a kidney transplant. Albuminuria (proteinuria) is also a risk factor for cardiovascular disease. Chronic kidney disease, of any cause, raises your cardiac risk and some doctors advise that statins are used if this is diagnosed.

Raised blood sugar levels can cause a rise in the degree of some chemicals in the kidney, which makes the glomeruli more leaky than normal and they scar the kidneys, which leaves the kidneys less able to filter the waste products out of blood.

Nerve damage (diabetic neuropathy) results when high levels of sugar in the blood over time stop our nerves from sending signals from your limbs (especially your legs and feet) to your brain. It can also affect the nerves in your body which control your heartbeat, which can make you more at risk of a heart attack and affect your digestion and your blood pressure.

Damage to the nerves which affect your arms and legs can result in numbness in the limbs, pins and needles, discomfort and shooting pains. It can also mean that you can damage your feet without realising it because of the loss of feeling – and this can, in turn, result in infections.

Eye problems. High blood sugar levels can cause problems with the eyes because they damage blood vessels in the eyes. This damage can cause problems such as retinopathy (damage to the blood vessels in the retina), cataracts (clouding of the eye's lens) and glaucoma - the buildup of fluid pressure inside the eye which damages vision. In the US, for instance, diabetes is the leading cause of blindness in American adults[6].

Gum disease. When you suffer from diabetes, the structure of your blood vessels is altered which affects the efficiency of the blood flow. This, in turn, may weaken the bone and the gums, leaving them more prone to infections. Also, you may have higher levels of glucose than is standard in the fluids of your mouth which can encourage the growth of gum disease causing bacteria.

Gum disease which is not treated and managed properly can result in tooth loss – and gum disease leads to high blood sugars, so it's a double whammy of a situation. Bacteria entering the blood stream from gum disease also cause worsening of heart disease.

Erectile dysfunction. To get an erection, men need healthy blood vessels, nerves, male hormones and desire. Because diabetes can damage the blood vessels and nerves which control the erection, a man can find himself either unable to get an erection or unable to sustain it in order to have sex.

Okay, so that is the doom and gloom of diabetes and poor blood sugar level control. And yet complications can be minimised, reduced completely, or even reversed by good enough blood sugar management[7].

The US Diabetes Control and Complications Trial (DCCT) which took place from 1983 to 1993 and the United Kingdom Prospective Diabetes Study (UKPDS – date 1977 to 1997) have firmly established that the better your control of blood sugar, the more likely you are to reduce your risk of complications from diabetes.

For insulin users, the downside to better control was that it also resulted in more frequent and more severe hypoglycaemia attacks. For patients with type 1 diabetes, and for the increasing number of patients with type 2 diabetes on insulin, this worry about hypoglycaemia has been a barrier to the introduction of more intensive treatment of diabetes. But at the time of the study, the connection was not made between the high amounts of dietary carbohydrates that were recommended to diabetics and the risk of hypoglycaemia.

Normal blood sugars without an excess of hypoglycaemia have been proven by the use of a controlled carbohydrate diet in conjunction with appropriate insulin techniques. Indeed, in a study carried out by Dr Jorgen Vesti- Neilsen, the renowned Swedish Diabetologist, there were 20 times fewer hypos on a low carbohydrate diet compared to baseline in type 1s in the first three months[8]. Furthermore, added benefits on weight control, blood pressure, triglycerides and high-density lipoproteins (HDL), which are the markers for metabolic syndrome and increased cardiovascular risk, are also improved on a carbohydrate-controlled diet[9].

In 2003 Jacqui Troughton, a specialist dietician at Warwick University in England, said that:

"Nutritional advice that has little or no supporting evidence is still being given to people with diabetes. People with diabetes need evidence based information about carbohydrates and to be given the knowledge and skills necessary to adjust their lifestyle, medication or insulin around the choices they wish to make."

(Troughton, 2003 Quoted in Practical Diabetes International).

Thankfully, the new evidence-based Scottish Intercollegiate Guidelines published in 2010[10], swept away the recommendation for the commonly used, high-carbohydrate, low-protein and low-fat diet for type ones and gestational diabetics. Advice for type 2 diabetics has broadened considerably to include lower total carbohydrate and lower glycaemic diets.

The American Association of Clinical Endocrinologists were the first body to recommend restricted carbohydrate diets for diabetics of all types from 2011 onwards. The Royal College of General Practitioners awarded their Innovator of the Year award to Dr David Unwin, who has promoted low carbohydrate diets in his England General Practice in 2016. The NICE Diabetes Guideline of 2016 does not promote any particular diet, but their criteria on what any proposed dietary advice should be based are met by the restricted carbohydrate diets that we describe in this book.

What this book is going to teach you is about what you can do to achieve better blood sugar levels – improving your life expectancy and the quality of your life right now. By eating mainly unrefined, minimally processed foods and matching your medication more precisely to your meals you can avoid the damaging blood glucose spikes that are known to cause ageing of all the tissues of the body, vascular changes, and adverse blood lipid patterns that cause the complications of diabetes.

The extent to which you may wish to achieve control over your blood sugars will vary. It is you the patient, or you the carer, who has to bear the physical and emotional burden of diabetic complications. We offer detailed advice on what long term blood sugar targets best meet your particular needs.

The choice of how far to restrict carbohydrates, and how tight the glycaemic control should be, is a decision that ethically remains with you. You will certainly have lots of options that will improve your control even if you don't take carbohydrate restriction to extremes or take up every insulin trick in the book.

CHAPTER SUMMARY

1. Diabetes is a life-long condition which can put you at risk of all kinds of complications, ranging from kidney disease to heart disease, blindness, nerve damage, gum disease and erectile dysfunction.

2. The easiest way to avoid these problems is to aim for excellent blood sugar control, as medical research has shown this to work and great blood sugar control CAN be achieved through matching insulin precisely to meals and eating mainly unrefined and unprocessed foods.

CHAPTER 2

WHY LOW FAT/HIGH CARBOHYDRATE DIETS DO NOT WORK FOR THOSE WITH DIABETES

Let's start with advice that no doubt most of you in the UK will already be familiar with – the "Eatwell" diet plate intended to show you what all health-conscious people and all diabetics, in particular, should be eating. One third of the plate is bread, rice, pasta and other starchy carbohydrates.

A diagram with the same sort of information is also given to the populace in the USA. The USDA food recommendations, though, say one quarter of the plate should be grains, and they specify wholegrains.

So, what is so wrong with this advice? Let's look at the problems with eating such a diet if you are diabetic. The UK plate recommends that meals should be made up of roughly:

1. a third of bread, rice, potatoes and pasta (items high in carbohydrates)

2. a third made up of fruit and veg (again, certain vegetables and fruit can be very high in carbohydrate)

3. a sixth of meat, fish, eggs and beans (beans and legumes can be high in carbohydrates)

4. a sixth of milk and dairy (certain dairy products contain relatively high amounts of carbohydrates, such as milk and flavoured yoghurt).

Why does a low-fat, high-carbohydrate diet such as the one set out by these examples NOT work for diabetics (type 1 and type 2s)? In Chapter 1, we looked at what diabetes is and why high blood-sugar levels in the body have such adverse effects, associated with all kinds of nasty complications such as heart disease, stroke, kidney problems and blindness.

The treatment of type 1 diabetes in the years before the discovery of insulin therapy in 1922 involved starvation – a diet which was extremely low in calories and carbohydrates.

This 'treatment' did not ultimately work, but it did extend the life of the children and young people diagnosed with the condition because it meant that they were consuming very few carbohydrates.

Carbohydrates raise the levels of sugar in the blood, which requires the action of insulin to convert that sugar into energy for the cells of the body. If insulin isn't present (as it is not in type 1 diabetics) or it does not work properly (as is the case with type 2s) then the sugar circulates in the blood and does damage to just about everything inside your body – your internal organs, your nerves and even your skin.

Common advice for people with diabetes is to avoid obviously high sources of sugary carbohydrates such as cakes, sweets, puddings, biscuits, and sugary drinks such as coke. But what about the supposedly slower-acting carbohydrates, seemingly "healthy" carbohydrates, such as wholemeal bread, brown rice, potatoes, fruit, beans and the other recommendations of the so-called healthy "Eatwell" plate?

All carbohydrate-containing foods will be broken down by the body into sugars, and all need to be dealt with by insulin that either your body produces or supplied medically. The more carbohydrates in the food eaten, the more insulin is required, but taking large doses of insulin to cover significant amounts of carbohydrates does not work precisely – as we will cover in Chapters 4, 5 and 6.

Starchy items are the backbone of the "Standard American Diet" and the diet that has been touted as the most heart healthy since the 1970s onwards. Unfortunately, all we have seen since starch has replaced fat is an increase in obesity, diabetes, heart disease and cancers.

For people with diabetes, it is madness to base meals around starch. If you eat meals based on starch, blood sugars rise, insulin increases (if you are still capable of producing insulin), and oxidative stress rises. Insulin resistance and then leptin resistance follow[11].

The body develops all the features of metabolic syndrome such as a big belly, high blood pressure, higher triglycerides, lower HDL levels (HDL is known as the "good cholesterol"), higher insulin levels and greater inflammation generally. All of these features are NOT just due to middle age, and they are not due to high-fat diets on their own. They are due to too much sugar and starch in the diet and all the features of metabolic syndrome can be reversed on a low carbohydrate diet[12].

Starch features prominently in both UK and USA diets, but there is absolutely no nutritional need for it. Any extra vitamins and minerals it has in it have been added back artificially. Think of the number of mass-produced breakfast cereals, for example, which boast of added vitamins and minerals in the attempt to persuade parents that they are buying a "healthy" choice for their children.

THE PROBLEM WITH GRAINS

Starch found in bread, pasta, potatoes, and breakfast cereals do fill people up and are relatively cheap.

The cheapness of starch is why it features so prominently in fast food – the buns, potato chips and dough balls which accompany burgers, or are side dishes for your pizza order (a particularly nasty double starch offering).

The problem is that these items are very high in carbohydrate, they tend to be addictive, and they do nothing for you, health wise. Grains, in particular, can interfere with the absorption of minerals from the gut and wheat is the number one food allergen.

Coeliac disease[13] represents one extreme of wheat/gluten intolerance, where sufferers must be vigilant in the avoidance of wheat in its many forms, but many more people suffer from irritable bowel symptoms, lethargy and general ill health while consuming wheat. All dramatically improve on stopping it.

Why the UK has a specific guideline advising that highly processed, high carb, high sugar, high salt, industrial fat containing junk is a reasonable part of a healthy diet is beyond silliness.

Highly-processed, high-carb, high sugar, high salt and industrial fat foods have unfortunately become a part of our standard westernised diets. They lead to addiction and ill health. The long working hours culture in the UK and USA are no doubt factors.

As women tend to work outside the home nowadays, processed food has filled a gap (and we are by no means criticising women for this, seeing as we are both female...). The problem is that your health is at stake here. There are enough meals that you can make from readily available items that would be better for you. Even more satisfying is learning to cook and bake the low carb way – and once you learn which foods to avoid, it is easy to adapt many of your favourite recipes to low carbohydrate, as we will show you in Appendix G.

From looking at the Eatwell plate again, you can see that certain foods are beneficial to diabetics such as low starch vegetables, limited quantities of fruit, white meat, seafood, limited amounts of red meat, eggs, unsweetened yoghurt, nuts, limited quantities of legumes, extra virgin olive oil, butter, coconut oil, and flaxseed oil.

But many of the items diabetics are expected to eat, and particularly in large quantities such as starch, are doing real harm.

THE BIG BAD EIGHT

The big eight foods to avoid on a diabetic diet are:

1. Fruit juice/sugary drinks
2. Sugar/ and sugar-containing items
3. Wheat/grains
4. Pasta/noodles
5. Potatoes/chips/crisps
6. Rice

7. Breakfast cereals, including porridge

8. Processed oils/margarines/processed food.

Why do you need to avoid the Big Bad Eight? **These foods make you feel awful. These foods make you hungry.**

When starch, fruit, fruit juice, sugar and sugar containing items are eaten, including the lactose present in milk, the sugars and starch are broken down into glucose and other sugars in the gut and absorbed by the stomach or intestine into the blood stream.

As far as your body is concerned it matters not one jot whether you have eaten a "healthy" baked potato or an "unhealthy" candy floss, it all ends up as sugar in the blood. Even higher fibre items get broken down into glucose. For instance, higher fibre breads become glucose only about 15 minutes later than white bread, and there are American studies which have shown that blood sugar levels rise higher after eating wholemeal bread than after eating candy bars[14].

When the glucose from these foods enters the blood, insulin is secreted from the pancreas to bring the blood sugar down. The glucose is taken up by receptors in muscle and tissue and used for making energy or glycogen. If not needed immediately it is stored as fat. All of this is supervised by insulin.

If you have early type 2 diabetes, insulin resistance syndromes (such as impaired glucose tolerance as it is called in the UK or pre-diabetes in the US), the glucose spike, quickly followed by an insulin spike can lead to more insulin than needed being secreted. This can give low blood sugars that in turn cause hunger – leading to more eating.

They cause tiredness.

The high glucose in the meal raises blood sugar. Although you may think that this should lead to you being more energetic, in fact, it leads to you feeling tired, sluggish and "can't be bothered". Ever had the feeling that you are too tired to talk, or that after a meal all you want to do is crawl into a corner of your office or home and sleep for a couple of hours? Welcome to post-prandial high blood sugars.

Your body works optimally at normal blood sugar levels (between 4 and 6mmol or 72-108mg), and high or low levels make you feel lousy.

Dr Morrison says: *"I used to feel exhausted, particularly after lunch. Fortunately, I would perk up at bit between 5-7pm before my evening slump. I didn't figure out it was what I was eating that was the problem until all this resolved on a wheat-free/low-carb regime."*

They make you fat.

Apart from the obvious correlation between eating carbohydrate, insulin secretion and the deposition of fat, there are longer term mechanisms at play that over time make you fat. In the short term, you can get away with eating almost anything, and you shouldn't get fat provided you stay within your body's caloric needs.

The issue here is insulin. Think of it as the boy who cried wolf. When insulin is secreted in high amounts over time (the boy keeps shouting wolf, and then keeps screaming it more loudly and more often as the townspeople ignore him) the body's cells become resistant to the message. The message of "wolf, beware!" is instead here, "body, take up glucose into the cell and burn it or store it". And the town folks (or the cells) are fed up of insulin continually shouting at them.

This leads to ever higher amounts of insulin being secreted to deal with the same glucose load. Insulin tells your body to store ingested carbohydrate as triglycerides. These raise fats in the liver, muscle and fat cells. These fat cells are also called adipocytes. From what you eat, a certain amount will start to be stored as fat and will not be available to be burned for energy.

CAN THE MIRROR LIE?

Insulin resistance leads over time to leptin resistance. Leptin is an essential hormone that governs appetite. The best explanation for this hormone comes from Byron J Richard's Mastering Leptin[15].

You know if you are fat or thin from looking in a mirror. Your brain, however, can't see. It "knows" if you weigh an appropriate amount by the level of leptin in the blood. If this is normal, your brain knows you weigh enough, and through leptin's effects on your stomach hormones (e.g. ghrelin), hunger is kept at bay.

If your brain is being told that you are too thin, it will affect hormones that will, in turn, increase your appetite. When your hormones are telling you to eat, you may be able to resist the urge for a time, but sooner or later you will eat.

Hormones are a bitch that way.

Skin infections and acne are worsened.

Bacteria and fungi just love sugar. High blood sugars make you less capable of fighting infection because the proteins on your immunoglobulins get glycated rendering them less effective.

Your skin, skin folds, nooks and crannies provide better surfaces for candida, tinea and bacteria, in general, to live off. If you are overweight, your skin folds become moist pockets where fungi and bacteria grow. Worsening acne, thrush, jock itch, intertrigo and athlete's foot occur more frequently and more severely if you have high blood sugars. These infections can be significantly reduced by losing weight and getting your blood sugar under control.

Are you feeling itchy yet?

They make you fat.

High-carbohydrate foods are addictive. Food manufacturers spend a lot of time and effort to make sure that you will eat their products and eat more of them when you do eat them – they are all desperately trying to bag up as much of your stomach space as they can.

Salt, sugar and fat and all kinds of artificial additives are added to make these foods more palatable and leave you wanting more – they go towards creating hyper-palatable foods.

OUR PERSONAL CARB TRIGGERS

Dr Morrison says: "Personally, I find that I really need to avoid Maltesers, cheese and onion crisps, Chilli Doritos and Sour Cream and Chive Pringles. Once I have a taste for them I just can't stop."

Emma says: "And I can't keep a particular brand of famous milk chocolate (the purple-wrapped stuff) in the house or any kind of cheese crisps. I am very partial to home baking, so I avoid keeping traditionally baked goods in my kitchen. If I don't have these things in the house, then the additional work of having to head out to a shop to buy them or having to bake cakes or biscuits from scratch puts me off. Sloth wins out over greed I suppose!"

Are you affected by these foods or is it something else?

Your body is never satisfied with starchy, sugary foods. People often report that they have room for sweet desserts, even if they feel full up before the dessert is offered.

Dr Morrison says: *"In the old days, before going wheat free and low carb, I used to have toast for breakfast, toast at 11am, a sandwich at lunch, a cake at 3pm, pasta with tomato sauce for dinner and cheese and crackers at 9pm. Every two or three hours I was looking for some other wheat/carb fix."*

They contain a lot of additives.

Read the ingredients of a ready meal when you are waiting on it coming out of the microwave. Do you know what half of the ingredients are?

We don't either. Maybe food scientists do. Ingredients in ready meals are often preservatives, salt, mono sodium glutamate, wheat, cheap fats, colourants, stabilisers or other such items; the kind of foods you don't have at home to add to the meals you make.

Do you know what is in a steak, an apple, a cauliflower and a handful of unsalted nuts?

Yes. Beef, apple, cauliflower and nuts. By keeping our food simple, we can retain some power over what we are putting into our bodies. Yes, if we want real control we might have to seek out organic products or meat and dairy products which come from grass-fed animals to minimise our contact with nasty pesticides and antibiotics. But even if you don't buy organic ingredients, it still beats the long list of what you see on a loaf of bread or a box of sweetened cereal.

Insulin sensitivity is worsened.

Sugar and wheat raise blood sugar, and eventually, insulin resistance occurs. This is the same way as saying that insulin sensitivity worsens. For type 2s, most of them reach this state quite gradually. In this condition, all of the features of metabolic syndrome develop. More medication is then needed to control blood sugar, blood pressure and lipids. Appetite and then weight become harder to control.

For type 1s, eating a high carb diet can eventually produce metabolic syndrome as well. This state is known as "double diabetes". Instead of needing one unit of rapid acting insulin to cover 10g of carbohydrate you may need one unit to cover a mere 3g. The worst example of this that Dr Morrison has seen was a type 2 woman using insulin who needed one unit to cover 0.5g of carbohydrate. Just for the record, an average apple contains roughly 15-20g carbohydrate so you can see that her insulin requirements were sky high.

These massive amounts of insulin then need to be injected. Absorption of insulin is not a precise science. Unless the seven-unit rule is followed (and we will give explanations of this rule in Chapter 4), the person is playing Russian Roulette with their diabetes control and will have unpredictable high and low blood sugar levels with each meal.

They raise blood sugar levels. They give you diabetic complications.

The main way that complications arise is the rise in blood sugar levels. The landmark US Diabetes Control and Complications Trial[16] (DCCT) proved that the higher the average HbA1c (a test routinely given to diabetics which looks at their average blood sugar level over a period of time), the more damage was done to the tissues of the body.

These adverse changes are known as diabetic complications. Some patterns of damage are individual to diabetes, for example, diabetic retinopathy and others mimic accelerated ageing of tissues such as arteriosclerosis and tendinopathy. The end result can be amputations, dialysis, blindness, chronic pain and digestive problems even to people in their 20s and 30s.

They encourage fat deposits in the liver.

The liver is the first port of call for the high blood sugars. Triglycerides are made here. Fructose, particularly concentrated fructose from high fructose corn syrup used in food manufacturing, is particularly problematical for causing fat storage in the liver[17].

This condition can worsen to cause fibrosis of the liver, also called cirrhosis[18]. Non-alcoholic fatty liver disease is now more widespread than its alcohol-induced counterpart.

In the future, it is thought that due to the growing "diabesity" epidemic that more transplants will be needed for this group of people. This problem can be prevented and reversed to some extent by weight loss and by adopting healthier eating practices[19]. A low-carb diet, which is low in sugar, starch, fructose and alcohol, can make a huge difference in recovery, provided cirrhosis has not yet occurred.

They glycate your proteins.

If you have high blood sugar levels, then the excess blood sugar molecules bind to cells and tissues of the body. The binding to red blood cells is the basis for the HbA1c test. Red blood cells live for about 120 days.

Measuring the level every two or three months can give a good reflection on what the average blood sugar levels have been over this period of time. When starting off on a low carb diet, it can be very encouraging to see this level drop dramatically. One type two patient of Dr Morrison's, for example, dropped from 17% to 7% in two months on a strict low carb diet of only 50g carbs a day. Some five years later her HbA1c is 6.0% just on her low carb diet and metformin 500mg twice a day. (IFCC 162 mmol/mol to 53 then 42)

Another body tissue that is prone to glycation is collagen. Collagen is usually arranged in layers like silk sheets gliding over each other. When extra sugar molecules bind bits of collagen together, the sheets become more like Velcro, and they stick to each other. Tendon movement then becomes restricted, and with Velcro-like collagen, you are more likely to get wrinkles and look old before your time.

They burst cells.

Sugar can become absorbed into some cells. The sugar molecules then attract water into the cell. These can then swell and burst. This is the basis of the nerve damage that is caused by diabetes.[20]

They encourage insulin dose stacking. They make managing your diabetes virtually impossible.

When you are eating a high carb/low-fat diet with not enough protein, you will usually feel hungry around every two to three hours.

What is worse is that you will probably be craving more carbohydrate to get that blood sugar up quickly. If you are using insulin, you will have covered your previous meal, but the insulin will still be active for several hours. You will need another dose of insulin and that dose still be working when your next main meal is due.

This leads to what is called "insulin stacking". It can be a cause of erratic blood sugars because you don't know precisely what is going on – is my insulin from the last meal still working or not? It is far better to eat nothing between meals unless you are covering exercise or treating a low blood sugar when it will be necessary to eat to stop the blood sugar levels dropping dangerously low.

When your next meal comes, you can give a correction dose of insulin if your blood sugar is a bit high, or give yourself less insulin for the next meal if your blood sugar is a little low. You will know where you are with your insulin and blood sugars much more than you will if you are eating every two or three hours.

High-carbohydrate foods are difficult to measure accurately.

Carb counting is an imprecise science. Packaging/carb counts can have errors of up to 20%[21]. Weighing is the most accurate way to do this, but you won't have your scales handy all the time. Can you imagine yourself, for example, taking weighing scales round to a friend's house and insisting on weighing out the potatoes he or she is serving you? Popularity among friends may not ensue!

When tested there can be about a 50% error rate in carb counting even when people have been taught the skills[22]. If you add in the insulin estimation necessary to cover those carbs, there can be errors here too.

You need high doses of insulin to cover large amounts of carbohydrate, and this is not absorbed predictably[23].

Absorption of this dose can have 30% variability unless you obey the seven-unit rule (which we explain fully in Chapter 4). The most efficient way is to eat low quantities of carbohydrate, use low amounts of insulin to cover the low-carb meal, eat when the previous dose of insulin is almost done, and inject in amounts of not more than seven units for each shot[24].

They cause low blood sugars.

A side effect of striving to cover high amounts of carb in the diet is low blood sugars. This is particularly common in the adolescent age group.

In the DCCT trial, teenagers had a 1% higher HbA1c than the adults in the intensive group and yet had a three times increased rate of hypoglycaemia that needed treatment from another person or hospital admission[25]. This is largely because of the severe insulin resistance that dominates the teenage years.

The peak for insulin requirement is aged 12 for girls and 14-16 for boys[26]. The blood sugar swings in a high carb diet are like massive ocean waves crashing up and down. The blood sugar swings on a low carb diet are more like ripples in a stream. And unless you like to live your life with diabetes like a surfer, you probably just want to cope with ripples.

In the DCCT trial, the average amount of carbohydrate consumed was 40% of calories. This works out as about 1,000 calories in a 2,500-calorie diet. Now diabetics have been urged to eat 55-65% of their energy from carbohydrates, which works out as 1,375 to 1,625 calories. No wonder diabetes control has seen no improvement in decades.

They cause beta cell death.

Beta cells that make insulin in the pancreas start to die off when blood sugars go over 5.6mmol/l (100 US)[27] . They recover when the blood sugars go lower, so the effect is to some extent reversible. When, however, they are subjected to high blood sugars for months on end, they die off permanently.

By the time a person is diagnosed with glucose intolerance, the precursor to type 2 diabetes, they have lost 10%-20% of their beta-cell mass. When a person is diagnosed with type two diabetes at least 50% of the beta cell mass have died[28]. By the time a type 2 diabetic needs insulin or a type 1 diabetic is newly diagnosed they have lost 80-90% of their beta-cell mass.

The apparent recovery that type 1s and 2s make when they are put on insulin is caused by the return to function of some of the beta cells from improved blood sugar levels. For type 1s this is called the honeymoon phase. It can usually last a few months to two years.

Some type ones who strictly low carb from diagnosis can last much longer than two years in this honeymoon phase.[29] If a type 2 diabetic starts to use insulin, they will usually get a considerable benefit from low carbing with much better blood sugar control with little or no hypoglycaemia for many years. In both cases, the background injected insulin is enough to do most of the work, and the remaining beta cells are providing a top up to order service that only a pancreas can do really well.

They raise inflammation levels. They give you cancer.

High inflammation levels are caused by high blood sugars which release oxidants into the tissues. This oxidative stress causes mutations in cells that can cause cancer[30].

Omega six oils found in processed seed and vegetable oils, margarine and processed food also cause high degrees of inflammation. These oils are associated with higher rates of cancer.[31]

By making you fat, they cause cancer. The risk of breast, endometrial, ovarian, kidney, thyroid, oesophageal, pancreatic, gall bladder, colon and rectal cancers are all raised the fatter you get[32] [33].

Raised blood sugars cause cancer. Your immune system is less efficient at policing rogue cells. Cancer cells thrive on sugar; it's what makes them multiply quickly.

They raise insulin levels and make you more likely to have a heart attack or stroke.

High insulin levels cause stiffening of the artery walls. This raises the blood pressure. The combination of stiffness and higher pressure aid the formation of small tears in the endothelium which lines the blood vessels. These then are plugged by the very small low-density lipoproteins (VLDLs) that are readily oxidisable[34].

These very low-density lipoproteins form plaques which can then rupture to cause a clot, which in turn can wholly or partly block a blood vessel anywhere in the body but most critically in the brain or coronary circulation[35].

They encourage oxidative stress.

Oxidative stress, in turn, affects endothelial function[36]. Arterial pressure rises after high carb meals due to changes to nitric oxide in the blood. There then occurs a chain reaction where cells are damaged by spare electrons looking for stability but causing havoc.

Oxidative stress is a no-no because it is linked with cancer, Parkinson's disease, Alzheimer's disease, heart failure, atherosclerosis, chronic fatigue syndrome and others[37].

Triglycerides are raised.

Triglycerides are deposited in the liver as fat and in fat cells. The fat cells, also known as adipocytes, produce inflammatory cytokines that affect hormonal systems in the body[38]. Metabolic syndrome features occur and worsen. Heart attack risk rises as triglycerides levels rise[39]. Dietary carbohydrate is the primary cause of raised triglycerides in the body, particularly carbohydrates of the refined variety[40].

HDL is reduced.

HDL is a type of lipoprotein, also known as "good" cholesterol, which is associated with longevity and the higher it is, the lower the heart attack risk.[41] The higher the level, the less cancer also tends to occur. Few things raise it, but the things that do are increasing naturally saturated fat in the diet,[42] reducing refined carbohydrates in the diet such as sugar and starch, and doing more exercise.

VLDL is increased.

Smaller, more readily oxidised VLDL particles are formed on high carb diets[43] . A marker for the benign bigger LDL particles which are not deposited in artery walls is a low triglyceride/HDL ratio. The ideal is under 1. Acceptable is under 2. At significant risk of arterial damage is 3.5 or above[44]. As an example, if your triglyceride levels are 0.5mmol and your HDL level is 2mmol then you have a ratio of 0.25 which is excellent.

High carb/low-fat diets do not improve long-term cardiovascular events.

The discovery that high-carbohydrate/low-fat diets (the standard weight loss/health improvement prescribed for many years) do NOT improve your chances of dodging a heart attack has been found in the Women's Health Initiative[45] (WHI) and the Multiple Risk Factor Intervention (MRFIT) trials[46], which looked at preventing heart attacks in men.

Therefore, in both genders, there is proof that these diets do not work. Also, further analysis of the WHI found that those in the intervention group had a worsened total mortality and cardiovascular mortality rate[47].

The Framingham study (a long-term heart health research project which began in 1948, testing out thousands of people from the town of Framingham in Massachusetts[48] only showed a benefit in reduced cholesterol in men under 50. In all other groups, total mortality improved on higher saturated fat and higher cholesterol levels.

High blood sugars interfere adversely with apo-lipoprotein a and b.

Lipoprotein a and b are blood markers that get less publicity than cholesterol, but in scientific circles, they are thought to be a much more reliable indicator of cardiovascular health than LDL cholesterol[49].

They cause abnormalities in the developing baby.

Dr Lois Jovanovich[50] and Dr C A Major have published papers showing that abnormalities in the developing baby can be PREVENTED by following a strict to moderate low carb diet[51].

Meanwhile, in the UK, diabetic pregnant women are still told to base their meals around starch. They have four to five times the severe abnormality rate as a result, despite free health care, free drugs, intensive treatment with pumps, increased monitoring and usually earlier deliveries in specialist units to pre-empt placental failure. Despite careful monitoring and liberal termination of pregnancy laws in the UK, the number of babies born with severe abnormalities to women with diabetes is double that of their non-diabetic sisters.

The main problem is that the high/low blood sugar swings cannot be prevented by a high carb diet. The strict levels of blood sugar control and an HbA1c level of under 6% are only achievable on a low carb diet. Dr Lois Jovanovich and doctors who use her protocols even manages to get her pregnant patients to have HbAIcs of 5.3% or less. She uses insulin liberally to achieve this and provides patients with continuous blood sugar monitors to detect hypoglycaemia.

They give you memory problems and dementia.

Dementia is often thought of as the third type of diabetes. Alzheimer's is increased by insulin defects in the cell that prevents amyloid plaques being removed.

Another type of dementia, multi infarct dementia is caused by vascular damage. This kind of dementia is particularly common in diabetics. Both of these types of dementia can be slowed with medication, but they are not reversible.

In general, poor concentration and memory happen even in school students whose blood sugars are too high[52]. This is reversible, but poor grades can affect further education and career choices for the future. Non-diabetic adults also perform worse on cognitive testing if their blood sugars are higher than those with lower levels of fasting blood sugars or HbA1c.

HIGH BLOOD SUGARS AND YOUR WORKING LIFE

My diabetes has never put me at real risk in a work situation, but I'd like to share with a story from some years ago...

I had just started a new job as a press and PR manager, and during my first week in the job, I attended a meeting with some pretty high-profile people who were also involved with the work my new organisation was doing.

The meeting started in the morning and continued into the afternoon. As was fashionable and convenient at the time, it included a working lunch of sandwiches. I ate three of them – little ones too, not a standard sandwich made with two slices of bread.

Twenty minutes into the post-lunchtime meeting and I was struggling to keep my eyes open as my poor body coped with blood sugar levels and insulin battling it out, with the result that blood sugar was moving around dramatically.

Granted, it was a mind-bogglingly dull meeting which could have been wrapped up well within an hour, but I couldn't even fake interest and, as for making a contribution to it and impressing my new boss – well, I was too busy concentrating on trying to keep my eyes open to do anything else. Speech was certainly not going to happen.

It's a relatively harmless example of what happens when poor concentration takes place thanks to those pesky high blood sugars, but many people with diabetes will be able to tell you the same story.

Added together, think of all of the opportunities we may have missed as a result – meaningful contributions to meetings, botched interviews, chances to shine avoided due to tiredness, tasks unfinished thanks to an inability to work...

(Low-carb) food for thought, hmm?

More drugs are required to control diabetes/complications/ co-morbidities

Higher doses of drugs and insulin are required on high carb diets. All drugs have side effects. The ACCORD trial was stopped prematurely as more deaths in occurred in the intensively managed group[53]. They had better blood sugar control due to taking more medications, but the side effects of drugs and hypoglycaemia were thought to be the cause of the worse outcome for these people.

You can control diabetes with a low carb diet and exercise far better than with drugs. Of course, you may still need some drugs and insulin, and certainly, that is the case for type one diabetes, but you will not need them to the same extent. Indeed, many people can considerably reduce their medications and insulin when they start a low carb diet.

High and low blood sugars interfere with driving safely.

Swinging high and low blood sugars are regulated by a low carb diet and worsened by a high carb diet. This is not helpful if you are driving. Concentration and reaction times are affected by both high and low blood sugars.

Accidents that have lethal or long-term effects on physical and mental health are a major issue for diabetics. If you can't drive, this can affect what work you are able to do and where you can do it. Good vision is also worsened by high blood sugars due to the effect of retinopathy, bleeds into the eye and macular degeneration.

So, there are all the reasons why a high-carbohydrate/low-fat diet is not a good idea for those with diabetes. Some reasons might be obvious and some not so – perhaps the additional risk of heavy wrinkles was not something you expected? But let us now move on to one of the simplest and easiest ways you can improve your health – the low carbohydrate diet – and a detailed explanation of what this is.

CHAPTER SUMMARY

The so-called healthy low-fat, high-carbohydrate diet prescribed to children and adults with diabetes is not healthy at all, and increased levels of carbohydrates in the diet lead to all kinds of problems – they make you hungry, they make you tired, they affect your eyes, kidneys, heart and encourage fatty deposits on the liver. They also raise the risk of hypoglycaemia in insulin-users because of the unpredictability of insulin needed to cover carbohydrates in meals.

CHAPTER 3

WHAT EXACTLY IS A
LOW-CARBOHYDRATE DIET?

Goodbye potatoes, farewell pasta, bye-bye rice and so long bread...
That's a low-carb diet, right?

Right – and sort of not right. While bread, rice, potatoes and pasta are obvious carbohydrate sources, along with anything sweet such as cakes, biscuits and chocolates, excluding them does not tell the whole carbohydrate story. There are carbs and thus hidden sugars in all kinds of sneaky places...

If you buy a sauce from the shops, chances are it will either have been thickened with flour or sweetened with sugar, honey or glucose. Tinned soups tend to have high carbohydrate contents, thanks to potatoes or flour/starch added as a thickening agent, and then there are beans, legumes, fruit and certain starchy veg such as sweet potatoes, beetroot and parsnips. All contain carbohydrates, and all will affect your blood sugar levels.

The standard recommendations given to people with diabetes from Diabetes UK[54] and the American Diabetes Association[55] is to focus on low-fat foods, whole grains, beans and legumes, lean protein, vegetable oils and plenty of fruit and vegetables. Typical advice is to avoid saturated fats, use low-fat dairy, substitute beans and legumes for meat in recipes and cut down or cut out sugar when making puddings.

This can still add up to a high-carbohydrate diet. Cereal and skimmed milk with fruit for breakfast, a roll and vegetable soup for lunch, potatoes, salmon and vegetables, finished off with fruit salad for dinner and a snack of a cereal bar or bran crackers with low-fat cheese spread. That's a day of eating which theoretically follows the recommended guidelines of both these organisations and yet this can stack up to as many as 160g carbohydrates, even if your serving sizes are tiny[56].

You may have received advice about the glycaemic index (GI) of food – the equivalent rate at which different foods release their sugar content into the body. As a rough rule of thumb, glucose is measured at 100 and protein only foods such as beef work out as very low on the scale. You may have been encouraged to concentrate on the foods which are low on the GI, which is where the recommendations of eating brown rice instead of white or eating fruits such as berries rather than grapes, come from.

But the GI is not a precise science and a food's GI can be affected by different things such as eating the food item with fat or protein. The rate of sugar release from an apple will be lower if it is eaten with a handful of nuts than if eaten on its own. How it's cooked will also affect the rate of sugar release. Baked potatoes, for example, are higher up the GI scale than boiled new potatoes. Hot mashed potatoes release their glucose even faster than the sugar you put in your coffee or tea.

CARBOHYDRATE COUNTING IN DAYS OF OLD

Years ago, I [Emma Baird] was taught a crude carbohydrate counting system based on exchanges – an exchange was roughly 10g of carbohydrates, and it was the way you used to count up the number of carbohydrates you were eating a day and match your insulin dosages to this.

Based on this system, an apple or an orange was roughly one exchange, so was a slice of bread and so was a heaped tablespoon of mashed potatoes or rice. The system had its merits, especially since the generation that came after me was not taught any form of carbohydrate counting at all. This seems to me to be almost criminally irresponsible. But old-style carb counting was based on post-war portion sizes. We hadn't been supersized then, but we certainly have now!

Industrial agriculture increased the size and sweetness of fruit. That 10g carbohydrate apple, for instance, no longer exists unless you grow your own. The apple you buy in the supermarket is more likely to work out as two if not two and a half times the number of carbohydrates and they go into your blood stream FAST.

Then there are bread sizes. Many modern day sliced loaves of bread are thick sliced and whole grain/multi-seed or not, two slices of these for a standard sandwich is likely to come in at 35-40g of carbohydrate.

Calculating the precise carbohydrate content of meals is much easier when the amount is small, and it makes eating out a much simpler and enjoyable experience.

Order a steak without the potatoes or chips and ask for extra veg and salad and you don't need to worry about weighing out the potatoes to calculate the carbohydrate count. This is not the easiest thing to do in a restaurant…You are also less likely to get post-meal hypos, thanks to too much insulin or high blood sugars thanks to too little.

The reasons given for NOT following a low-fat, high-carbohydrate diet in the last chapter may well have convinced you that it can help you towards better blood sugar levels, better HbA1 results, a general improvement in energy and a decreased risk of diabetes-related complications, but "low-carbohydrate" can strike fear into the uninitiated:

1. What will I eat?
2. It's all bacon and eggs for breakfast for ever more…
3. But I LOVE bread and cakes, what will I do?
4. What about constipation/nutrients/my cholesterol levels/XYZ – [insert your concern of choice]

We hope to address your concerns throughout this book and particularly in Chapter 9, the frequently asked questions (FAQs) section, but just to answer these four quickly:

You can eat plenty.

You don't have to eat bacon and eggs for breakfast every day, though, for many people, including the authors of this book, that is a real treat and not a sacrifice.

Bread and cakes are a possibility as you will see from our recipe section at the back.

Constipation shouldn't be a problem. If it is, we tell you about how to deal with it in the FAQS.

There are various definitions of what counts as a low-carbohydrate diet. For the purposes of this chapter, think of the definitions as:

1. Very low carbohydrate, 50g or less
2. Moderate carbohydrate, 50-90g
3. Up to 130g of carbohydrates is still counted by some as low carbohydrate, as it is still a lot less than the average carbohydrate consumption where people eat bread, pasta, pizza, cakes or sweets.

The extent to which you may wish to achieve control over your blood sugars will vary. It is you the patient, or you the carer, who has to bear the physical and emotional burden of diabetic complications. The choice of how far to restrict carbohydrates, and how tight the glycaemic control should be, is a decision that ethically remains with the patient – or in other words, you.

What restricting carbohydrates can do is to give you greater control over your blood sugar levels. When you attempt to match insulin doses to the carbohydrate content of high-carbohydrate and low-fat meals – let's take as an example the bread roll and vegetable soup example given earlier – you run the risks of mistakes. A lunch of vegetable soup and a bread roll might contain 60g carbohydrates, or it might even total 100g of carbs, depending on what is in the soup, how large the roll is and what portion sizes you take – so you might match a meal with a large dose of insulin to compensate.

Guess what? Significant inputs cause BIG mistakes, whereas small inputs, the amount of insulin needed to cover a steak and vegetables, for example, cause small mistakes[57]. The results are 80-2,000% fewer hypos on a moderate carbohydrate regime of 70-90g,[58] [59] and the very low carbohydrate regime espoused by Dr Bernstein can lead to almost no hypos[60] (if you aren't doing a lot of exercise).

Let's look at what the different low carbohydrate diets mean...

VERY LOW CARBOHYDRATE REGIMES

Dr Richard Bernstein's diet for diabetics, as outlined in the Diabetes Solution and the Atkins induction phase of low carb dieting advocate a very low carbohydrate approach of under 40g of carbohydrates a day, with the Atkins diet recommending 20-30g of carbohydrates a day. The Atkins induction phase sets out this low carbohydrate count initially so that dieters achieve nutritional ketosis[61], which should not be confused with ketoacidosis[62], which is very dangerous for type 1 diabetics.

Bernstein recommends a very low carbohydrate intake for people with diabetes permanently to achieve extremely tight blood sugar controls. As the carbohydrates in vegetables, even vegetables such as broccoli, cauliflower, lettuce and courgettes count, then doing a low carbohydrate diet this way mostly means eating a few vegetables, no grains, no beans or legumes and no sweet fruit. The calories in the diet are provided by protein, measured amounts of low carbohydrate vegetables and large quantities of fat.

This very low level of carbohydrate is recommended for those people seeking very tight blood sugar control – for example, women planning a pregnancy or to reverse diabetic complications such as neuropathy (nerve damage), retinopathy (eye problems) and kidney problems. It can almost eliminate hypos (low blood sugars), and it is suitable if you prefer to use very low doses of insulin, as your requirements for insulin will drop sharply when eating this way. It can give you an HbA1 level of 4.2 to 5.5% which is the kind of level people without diabetes experience, although it's hard for menstruating women to achieve levels of less than 5.0 % because of fluctuating hormone levels.

THE TROUBLE WITH HYPOS, Emma Baird

We keep talking about hypos (low blood sugars) in this book, but what exactly are they and why do they cause problems?

As so much of our health depends on preventing the problems resulting from high blood sugars in the body — they raise your triglyceride levels, which is implicated in the increased risk of heart disease, and high blood sugar levels are toxic to almost every organ in the body, as well as affecting nerves, your eyes, your skin and your joints — it might be tempting to think, "Well, low blood sugars, so what? That's good, hmm?"

Not so fast... As anyone on insulin or medications which stimulate insulin secretion will ever have experienced, hypos can be very unpleasant when they happen. Symptoms range from feeling weak and tired to being unreasonable and grumpy, as my husband could certainly tell you, moody and snappy, hungry, clumsy, sweaty and trembling. I even had a phase of crying whenever I was hypo, a most unwelcome development.

Just as untreated high blood sugars create havoc as they charge through the body, untreated low blood sugar levels (less than 3.9mmol or 70mg) will eventually deprive the brain of so much sugar that you faint or start fitting. Again, if you faint and treatment is not administered quickly, then you risk slipping into a coma or even dying. So good reasons to avoid hypos, don't you reckon?

Another problem with low blood sugars levels is what happens afterwards. If my blood sugar slips below 2.6mmol or 50mg, then it unleashes the most incredible hunger. This is when, as many people who have type 1 diabetes or who are on insulin-stimulating drugs will testify, you find yourself surfacing from a brain fog surrounded by empty sweet packets.

The standard treatment for a hypo is roughly 15- 20g of fast-acting carbohydrates such as three or four glucose tablets or jelly sweets, or a small glass of a sugary drink such as full-sugar Coke or Lucozade.

Eating a much larger amount of rapid-acting carbohydrates in one go will have a knock-on effect later. I once racked up an entire bag of jelly babies and several slices of bread because of very low blood sugar levels – taking in about 180g carbohydrates in just under 15 minutes.

From 2.6mmol (50g) to 22mmol (390g) – it really isn't a pleasant feeling.

The causes of hypos vary, but some of the common ones are: taking too much insulin; not eating enough food; doing a lot of exercise and drinking alcohol.

Eating a low carbohydrate diet reduces the risk of hypos because you will not need as much insulin to cover your meals and you will be able to lower your daily background dose.

MODERATE CARBOHYDRATE INTAKES

Next up is the more moderate low carbohydrate option of around 50-90g a day, which is rather easier to follow than a very low carbohydrate option because it allows for a little more food choice.

We will go into sample menu plans for both low and moderately low carbohydrate diets later in this book, but to give you a rough idea, on a moderate carbohydrate intake you can:

1. add in fruit (though many fruits are high in carbohydrates, so the encouragement is to stick to fruits such as berries, citrus fruits, plums, apricots and pears and only 1-2 servings a day)

2. broaden the selection of vegetables you are using

3. add in small quantities of whole grains or beans and legumes if you like.

Swedish diabetologist Dr Jorgen Vesti Nielson trialled a 70-90g carbohydrate diet (i.e. 20% of the calories in the diet were provided by carbohydrates[63]) over almost four years at his Blekingesjukhuset Clinic. As a result of his trial, the average HbA1 result for type 1 diabetics was 6.4% (without the advanced insulin techniques we describe in this book), and type 2 diabetics were 5.8%.

In his study of a low-carbohydrate diet[64] tested out on people with type 2 diabetes, Nielsen noted that a significant effect was the absence of hunger when restricting carbohydrates to 20% of the diet. His 44-month study showed that lasting effects on body weight and blood sugar control results from this more moderate carbohydrate reduction.

For such a diet, you will need carbohydrate counting skills to precisely work out what you are eating, and you will need to know how to match your medications to this level of carbohydrates. You will need to weigh and measure a lot of what you are eating, and the bulk of your calorie intake will still come from fat. Just as with a very low carbohydrate diet, high amounts of protein in the diet can cause blood sugar levels to rise.

LOW-CARB EATING = DRAMATIC RESULTS by Dr Katharine Morrison

I have been advocating low carb diets for those patients with impaired glucose tolerance, metabolic syndrome, type two diabetes and type one diabetes for more than fourteen years now.

The most dramatic drop in HbA1c was in a newly-diagnosed type 2 diabetic of 47 years of age who went from an HbA1c of 17% to 7% in two months, only taking Metformin 500mg at night as an adjuvant drug. Her HbA1c is 6.0% six years later with no additional medications. (IFCC 162 to 53 then 42)

My best successes for the lowest HbA1c without hypos have been 4.8% both in insulin users. (IFCC 29)

One was a 60-year-old type 2 diabetic woman who chosen to follow a low-carb diet and use insulin after reaching an HbA1c of 11.8% on maximal oral drug therapy for years. She has maintained the level of 4.8% for six years now.

The other was my son who was a newly diagnosed type 1 diabetic, whose pancreas recovered somewhat after starting insulin and a low carb diet from the time of diagnosis in 2004. As his pancreas failed, this level (4.8%) gradually increased, and his HbA1c was 5.8% some ten years later. Now that he lives alone in his own flat and drives a car, his blood sugar targets are little higher, and his HbA1c is 6.0%. (IFCC 29 in honeymoon to 40 then 42)

I have met other diabetics, mainly type 1 men who have reached HbA1c of 4.2% on Dr Bernstein's low carb diet and through using a highly-advanced insulin regime and regular weight training. (IFCC 22)

How to use insulin and low-carb eating to achieve lower HbA1cs is discussed in this book, but Dr Bernstein's own textbook, The Diabetes Solution, goes into much more detail for those who wish to really nail their blood sugars. Menstruating women find it impossible to achieve these results due to hormonal fluctuations and the best they usually manage is a percentage higher than this at 5.2-5.5%. (IFCC33-36)

However, women are very unlikely to get diabetic complications with HbA1cs of 5.5% and under, and they just have to accept that this is the case, just as most women will find that men tend to find sticking to diets easier and lose weight on them more quickly as well. (IFCC 36)

My "average" patient tends to have a starting HbA1c of 8.5-9.5%, and many of them get to HbA1c of 5.5-6.5% on a "moderate" low carb diet of around 60-90g of carb a day plus regular exercise. What is more, the results are seen very quickly. Blood sugars revert to near normal within hours to days. (IFCC 69-80 on average dropping to 36-47).

In this chapter, we have outlined the definitions of low carbohydrate diets and their reported benefits on your blood sugar levels, but what are the other benefits you can expect?

Stable blood sugar levels mean steady levels of energy through the day. This might not sound like a biggie, but if you spend your days wanting to take a nap after meals, it can make a huge difference.

Weight loss. As reported earlier, Dr Nielsen's study showed the positive effects of a low-carbohydrate diet on diabetic patients' weights. Weight loss in people usually occurs for two reasons – lower blood sugars mean the body is not forced to dump excess sugar levels in cells resulting in fat and weight gain. Secondly, a low-carbohydrate diet naturally decreases hunger and increase satiety when eating, often resulting in people eating less not because they think they should, but because they just don't want to.[65] If you are someone who has battled with will power all your life, this is brilliant news.

Better sleep. Again, steady blood sugars mean better quality sleep as the body isn't battling high or low blood sugar levels as you sleep.

Reversal of diabetic complications. This takes a long time, but Dr Morrison has seen this happen in her practice.

REVERSING COMPLICATIONS by Dr Katharine Morrison

One of my type 2 patients had a chronic foot ulcer that was not healing, despite in-patient treatment in hospital and lots of antibiotics over 18 months. He wanted to avoid an amputation, and this seemed increasingly likely.

He went on a strict low carb diet, and the ulcer started to heal within days. It cleared up, and he got no more ulcers over the next five years. The pain and numbness also reversed over this period of time.

Another type 2 patient was getting laser treatment to his eyes every two months over at least a year. He went on a low-carb diet and, at his next visit to the hospital, the ophthalmologist said, "What have you done?" "I'm on a low-carb diet," he replied. "Well, carry on with it, because you have stopped bleeding into your eyes".

This patient did not need any further laser treatment over the next four years when he moved away. His retinopathy went into reverse, and his optician and ophthalmologist reported gradual improvement every time he saw them. Although he never obtained useful eyesight in his bad eye, the vision improved very gradually in his other eye.

Other reported benefits include better skin, better digestion, better hair and nails – oh and a much flatter stomach. Aesthetic considerations may not be your primary goal (and if this is so, we salute you!) but a flatter stomach thanks to the loss of midriff fat is a side effect of low-carbohydrate diet and one that we reckon most people will welcome.

This chapter has outlined the basics of low-carbohydrate eating, but before we start describing what you can and cannot eat, the next few chapters are going to teach you in-depth about managing your medication on a low-carbohydrate diet. Low-carbohydrate dieting will change your life for the better – but if you know the exact skills you need for managing your medication, prepare for your life to change entirely forever and for you to achieve results you never dreamed were possible...

CHAPTER SUMMARY

Low-carbohydrate diets can vary from as low as 30-40g to up to 130g of carbohydrates a day. The lower the carbohydrates, the more likely you are to achieve tighter blood sugar control and better HbA1cs, but this is an individual decision. Low-carbohydrate diets, in general, involve eating meat, fish, eggs, some dairy, non-starchy vegetables, limited fruit and healthy fats, and they can result in better blood sugar results, increased energy, reversal or halting of diabetic complications and weight loss.

CHAPTER 4

SUCCESS STORIES

Seeing how other people have worked to better their health, and the success they have achieved thanks to changing their diet can really spur you on to make the necessary changes to your own diet and life.

Here, a few people explain why changing to a low-carbohydrate diet worked for them...

James' Story:

I managed to lose four and a half stones in weight and bring my blood sugars under control after I started to follow a low-carbohydrate diet of 60-80g carbs a day and I used the medication prescribed.

This was managed after consultation with and continued monitoring by Dr Morrison. Before starting this, I was already on Metformin 500mg three times a day with meals and a statin once a day. I continued with this but used it in conjunction with a Byetta 5mls injection morning and night before meals.

After reaching my target weight, I stopped taking the Byetta, and I subsequently elected to also stop the statin. I am now only taking Metformin, and I use this in conjunction with the low carbohydrate diet supported by regular testing with strips when required.

If, while monitoring, I find that my blood sugars are higher than usual I am able to adjust by dropping the carb intake or through more exercise. Thanks to this combination, I am able to keep on top of my weight and blood sugars. Being able to test regularly is an important safety net which helps to keep things on track.

Before this, I was following a standard diet sheet issued to diabetics which recommended numerous suggestions that were high in carbohydrates. Even with regular exercise using the diet sheet in conjunction with the Metformin I was not able to lose the weight, and my blood sugars were not consistent.

While following both the previous regimes I was able to carry out regular exercise as we run a small holding with numerous animals.

Before I lost the weight, I was unable to carry out more than about half an hour of work before I needed to rest. I was regularly out of breath. Now I can work on to suit myself and don't feel limited as much by diabetes.

Sandra's Story:

I am 68 years old, and I was diagnosed with type 2 diabetes 12 years ago.

My initial blood glucose readings were very high, and I was feeling very unwell. All I wanted to do was sleep, and I could not stop drinking fizzy drinks. With the help and advice from my Diabetic Care Team, I went on a controlled diet and exercised daily.

I went for diabetic reviews twice a year, and all was fine. I was keeping good control of my blood sugars.

After about three years, I was diagnosed with osteoarthritis in my knee. I had a knee replacement in 2006 and could not exercise as much as I had been doing.

I also had high blood pressure, and it took a few months to get it under control (I now take medication for it).

But I was also having a big problem keeping my blood sugar under control at this time.

My GP, a Dr Morrison, worked very closely with me and suggested a low carbohydrate diet. I made changes to what I was eating and found that in a short time I was feeling a lot better and my blood sugar was under control again.

I no longer eat foods that are high in carbs I now eat lots of grilled fresh fish, chicken, lean steak, veg, fruit, eggs, and lots of salads, I drink lots of water as I don't drink tea or coffee and no longer eat any processed food at all.

(I do allow myself a treat now, and then, such as when I go out to dinner I will have a sweet.)

I take medications called Metformin and Sitagliptin each day. I found that with the low-carb diet and moderate exercise I have been able to keep my blood sugars under control.

And I must say I feel a lot better since eating low carbohydrate food.

Ron's Story

Ron Raab OAM, B.Ec has had type 1 diabetes for more than 55 years, and he has written and advocated extensively in favour of a low-carbohydrate, moderate protein and healthy fats approach to the treatment of diabetes.

He is the president of Insulin for Life (IFL) Australia and IFL Global (www.insulinforlife.org) an organisation which donates in-date and no longer needed insulin and other supplies to countries in need. He was also a Vice President of the International Diabetes Federation.

I was diagnosed with type 1 diabetes in 1957 at the age of 6. I had the typical program of urine testing, animal insulin and then in 1980, self-blood glucose monitoring, and then the use of "human" insulins.

In my view, the 1980s were a particularly dark period in the evolution of diabetes dietary recommendations. Why? The change to the high carbohydrate (CHO) recommendations have been a disaster for diabetes treatment and have also been a major contributing cause of the diabetes epidemic.

Diabetes is essentially a disorder of CHO metabolism/ intolerance. High CHO recommendations make excellent moment-to-moment blood glucose impossible. They require high insulin doses, and it is also impossible to measure carbohydrates accurately or be able to closely predict the absorption profiles of carbohydrates and insulin.

In the early 1990s, I "saw the light" and began to eat a low carbohydrate regime under professional guidance. There is a great deal of interest and implementation by people with diabetes of this regime; but the mainstream advice by diabetes organisations and health professionals does not reflect this, even though basic physiology and evidenced-based research do. The result is that many people with diabetes miss out.

Essentially, a low carbohydrate regime means much less insulin is needed, and this results in vastly improved moment to moment blood glucose levels. At the same time hypos and particularly serious hypos decrease. My HbA1c improved dramatically, and overall I felt much better and have been able to maintain this.

The current recommendations overlook a fundamental reality: blood glucose levels in people with diabetes vary with increasing unpredictability as the consumption of carbohydrate increases. A low intake of carbohydrates requires smaller amounts of insulin, resulting in increased predictability and much smaller variation in blood glucose levels.

Graeme's Story

I was diagnosed with type 2 diabetes in 2002 at the age of 61, and my GP prescribed Metformin to help lower my blood sugars.

I was shocked by the diagnosis as I'd always been fit, healthy and active, but my great grandmother had died from the side effects of diabetes complications of 46, so I thought it must have been genetic.

I'd been given a guidebook by my GP about how to live with the condition, and I wondered if there might be a way of dealing with my diabetes without using drugs. I knew nothing about diabetes and had no medical knowledge, but as a businessman, I'd spent my working life analysing and dealing with problems, so this was just another problem to solve.

The guidebook I had received from my GP suggested a diet which included starchy foods such as rice, potatoes and pasta, but I soon realised that if I followed this advice that I would be unable to control my blood sugars without taking medication. I bought myself a blood glucose testing kit, and I tested my sugar levels six times a day. I started graphing the results, and I soon realised that changes in my sugar levels related directly to what I was eating, so I began to cut out the foods which were pushing my blood sugar levels above normal – such as pasta, rice, potatoes, bread and sugary foods.

Within a year, I had given my diet a complete overhaul, and I was eating lots of fish, shellfish, egg, meat, nuts, berries, leafy vegetables and herbs – basically the diet followed by our hunter-gatherer ancestors.

I did a bit of research online and discovered many other type 2 diabetics who had followed a similar diet and achieved success. But in January 2005, a routine check-up revealed my HbA1c was 7.1% and my GP advised that I start on medication to stabilise my diabetes.

This time, I completely cut out cereal, bread, milk, red meat and dairy products and four months later, my HbA1c had fallen to 5.1. His HbA1c has risen in the last seven years, but it is still within the normal range.

To keep me going on the diet, I developed a low-carb bread which doesn't raise my blood sugar levels. I even take it with me when I go to hotels.

I believe that this way of treating diabetes does not get promoted because of the lack of studies. Most research comes from drug companies who are not interested in investigating whether there is a way to deal with diabetes without medication.

Vicky's Story

My daughter Vicky was diagnosed with type 1 diabetes in October 2011 at the age of seven.

While I was in the hospital with Vicky after her diagnosis, we were woken at 2am by a nurse with a bowl of apple crumble and custard. Vicky, of course, was delighted – the nurse's explanation was that Vicky had not had her recommended daily allowance (RDA) of carbs the previous day so this was a catch-up. I queried this with the consultant the next day - "why give a sugar-rich meal to someone with a sugar-based condition?". But the consultant just blamed RDAs.

We then decided that we needed to avoid sugars and starches. In addition, I have a potential heart problem, so I had begun to look into low-carb diets as the healthier option for me, if not the whole family.

The doctors and nutritionists did not know what a low-carb diet would entail, so we researched the issue ourselves. We debated – will this benefit us? How low is low? If we eat low-carb, what is the best mix regarding protein/fat and how will this work in real life for our family?

From our research, we concluded that low-carbing would benefit us. We set a maximum of 30g carbs a day, and we went for a diet high in natural fats. Dr Morrison put us onto low carb forums which gave us access to additional recipes. We did a big shop for the necessary ingredients, gave away the high carb foods we had in the house and read up on the recommendations from Dr Bernstein and Barry Groves.

We set up a regime of vitamins and minerals for Vicky (we all take them now). These include chromium, natural Vitamin E, Vitamin C, Evening Primrose Oil and niacinamide.

It would be a lie if we said it was a seamless process but it wasn't THAT difficult. It has been helped more so by the fact that, over time, my wife has perfected fabulous dishes in themselves as well as ones that replace things we missed or liked such as moussaka and pizza. She also makes her own low-carb cakes and biscuits. At first, she got the recipes from books and /or the internet forums. Now she makes her own ones up.

We have never had any problems with the school since the girls take in their own lunches, or with family, who love the recipes and food, or the girls' friends. For parties, they bring their own food. With three young daughters, we don't eat out too much, but when we do we explain what we want and how we like it. If they can't do it; we don't go there.

We found two things to be incredibly helpful when it came to cooking:

1. Stevia: we found a herbalist who compounded his own (Alan Hopking) which replaced sugar in more or less everything.

2. Ground Almonds: organic to replace flour. We got these off the internet and from Indian stores.

In addition, we try to eat organic food such as chicken, eggs and lamb as much as possible.

As a result of our diet, I have lost some 12kgs (26.5lbs or almost two stone), and this has remained off. The weights of our daughters and my wife have remained constant as none of them was overweight. We DO feel better for it. Okay, we miss the odd tempting smell of baking in shops, but we know that this is greatly outweighed by how we feel.

Vicky takes one injection of Levemir (basal insulin) a day in the morning of 5 units. Her last HbA1c was 5.8% (IFCC 36), and it was the same six months previously.

I am convinced that the life sciences world will find an approved medicine that is not insulin and not in injection delivery form in the next 5-10 years. I know a number of small and big pharmaceutical companies are well under way with their clinical trials

We will stick with the low carb framework we have, however, we are looking at two things: one is the acidity/alkalinity body levels which are almost entirely affected by food, and reducing our intake of meat while increasing our intake of vegetables/salads. Vicky has started a course of osteopathic manipulations and massages which is an old therapy. It will be interesting to see if there are any changes.

We are SO glad that we stumbled upon low carbing, which is truly part of how we live. We never knew just how important nutrition generally and food, in particular, is to our health and well-being. The outcomes speak for themselves.

I've offered to go through with the consultants and hospital nutritionists what we do so they can see if it can be used for other children and adults. Sadly, there has been no take-up of the offer yet.

Resources we found useful

- Atkins: `Quick and Easy New Diet Cookbook` [any Atkins book !!]
- Bernstein: `Diabetes Solution`
- Groves: `Trick and Treat` and `Natural Health and Weight Loss`

- Brighthope: `The Vitamin Cure for Diabetes`
- Kossoff et al.: `Ketogenic Diets.`

Emily's Story

I am 42, and I have type 1 diabetes, which I control through an insulin pump. I changed to an insulin pump six years ago because my needs for long-acting insulin were quite small and I was getting hypos twice a day. [Pumps only use one kind of insulin – a rapid acting one.]

My insulin needs vary considerably through the day, and I have been able to set my pump accordingly. I restrict my carbohydrates to 75g per day (20-25g per meal). On a pump, what I can do is take my bolus in one dose just as you would do with injections, or take it over a longer period of time. This is very useful for low carb/fatty meals.

I could choose to eat pizza and ice-cream from time to time if I wanted, but I only do so very occasionally.

On the pump I use, I have the option of three basal patterns [the basal pattern is the amount of background insulin going into you over the course of a day]. If I were going to be very active, for example, I would opt for a lower amount of basal insulin. This feature is also useful to prevent alcohol-induced hypos: I reduce my overnight basal to 90% to avoid night-time or early morning hypos. You can also reduce the basal percentage for some hours, which is great for exercise. It also helps to be able to control basal levels at different times of the menstrual cycle.

I would highly recommend pumping to anyone who has unexplained hypos on a regular basis.

I started low carbing because it was so obviously illogical to eat a high carb diet even when it is endorsed by the NHS and Diabetes UK. I wanted to get rid of post meal blood sugar spikes and also wanted to lose weight. I researched the diet, and I gradually reduced my carbs from 120-150g a day to 90g and then I aimed for 60-75g. My dietician said she didn't recommend going below 90g a day, but she couldn't explain why, so I ignored her and got down to 60g a day, but found this too difficult to maintain as I follow a vegan diet.

I am an expert in my own reduced carb, vegan diet and find using a pump makes it much easier to eat the diet that suits me and keeps my insulin doses low. My blood sugar levels are as good as they can be. For the past few months, I have also been doing the 5:2 fasting diet which is fine on a pump. On a pump, you can eat like a normal person – you can eat five small meals a day or two big ones, or you can fast. It's also easier to correct slight highs as you can give yourself tiny amounts of insulin.

If people want to go on a pump, I think they ought to research all the different companies and models available. Some hospitals are tied to particular makes of the pump, so find this out too. When weighing up options, you should consider the availability of a helpline number, the ordering process for supplies and the choice of infusion sets.

You also need good support when making the transition. I took a week off work, which I would highly recommend. You also need a good diabetes support nurse who you can call on to help you sort out all the teething problems you will experience in the first few days or weeks. In addition, one of the best places for finding out information about insulin pumping is through the website – Insulin Pumpers UK, as you can get so much advice and information from other people using pumps.

Steven's Story

I've had type 1 diabetes for ten years (I'm 22 now).

I felt tired and imbalanced when I was first diagnosed with diabetes. The diabetic clinic didn't advise me to follow a low-carbohydrate diet, but they did warn me to avoid sugars. I had been eating pizza, pasta, vegetables, cereal and other "normal" foods beforehand, but my mum put me on a low-carbohydrate diet when I was diagnosed.

Nowadays, I eat about 100g of carbs on a standard day, which includes adjustments for hypos and meals. I like that my diet includes lots of steak, chicken and bacon, though I do miss not being able to eat pasta and rice. As long as I keep my diet varied, it is pretty easy to follow. I'm delighted that my diet has kept me away from the potential side effects of diabetes and my last Hba1c result was 5.8%.

Lucy's Story

I don't have diabetes, but I did want to lose a bit of weight before my 40th birthday, and I offered to try out my sister's diet when she told me about it.

I did the diet for seven weeks. I do have four young boys, so I needed quite a few quick and easy options such as Greek yoghurt, berries and flaked almonds for breakfast. I also really liked the moussaka recipe. I lost 12 pounds in the seven weeks – taking me from 10 stone 3lbs at the start (143lbs) to 9 stone 5lbs (131lbs). It was a really easy diet because I didn't get hungry and I lost all my cravings for sweet foods and things such as crisps.

I noticed a lot of improvements to my health – I slept a lot better, I felt as if I had more energy and my digestion really improved. I noticed that I wasn't farting as much – my family could tell you that I've always been a bit of a farter!

I'll be keeping the diet up because it is so easy to follow and because I do feel so much better. I'll probably add in a few more carbs though, just to make it a bit more flexible.

Fergus's Story

I'm now 49, and I've had diabetes for 31 years since I was 18. My last HbA1C result was 4.8% (29 mmol).

When I was first diagnosed, I was thirsty and emaciated. When I was diagnosed, I was on essentially, a 'healthy' (by an NHS definition) diet. At the time I was vegetarian and so followed a diet naturally low in saturated fat, and based predominantly around starchy carbohydrate foods. Typical daily fare would include breakfast cereal, sandwiches, fruit, pasta, cheese, yoghurt etc. The diabetes clinic had never mentioned a low carbohydrate diet. Such dietary advice as I received was firmly based around starchy carbohydrate foods.

I decided to follow a low carb diet because I needed to lose some weight and reduce my HbA1c (at the time around 7-8%) but had little or no understanding of the mechanisms at work.

Once I realised that insulin levels were fundamentally linked to my body's ability to gain weight, it seemed obvious that reducing my weight would depend on reducing my insulin dose. In turn, the only way to do that without going hungry would be to eat the foods that demanded less insulin. After some experimentation, my insulin intake fell to around 25% of my previous needs, without giving much regard to my calorie intake!

Within a year, my excess weight had gone, my BMI was 22 and, the ultimate bonus, my HbA1 was below 5.0%. I've been on a low carb diet for 14 years now.

I eat 20-30 grams of carbohydrate daily, occasionally less. A typical day might include a cheese and mushroom omelette at breakfast, chicken or mackerel for lunch with a salad or some vegetables and dressing or mayonnaise, for dinner meat or fish with any number of vegetable choices, home-made low carbohydrate bread, cheeses, red wine, 85% cocoa chocolate. I drink black tea or coffee with cream throughout the day.

At first, I did miss some foods. I would miss pasta, potatoes and especially cheesecake. After a few weeks, however, these feelings subsided, and these days I really have no desire for them anymore.

I feel great on a low-carb diet. I cycle every day, sometimes long distances when the weather permits. One of the pervasive myths that has attached itself to low-carb diets is that carbs are essential for physical exercise, but that has never been my experience. Quite the reverse, in actual fact.

I have no diabetic complications at all, despite having the condition for almost a third of a century. Oh my god, have I really been type 1 for that long? My HbA1c has remained between 4.5 and 5% at every visit to my diabetic clinic for over a decade. The clinicians were certainly sceptical when I explained how I achieved that, but I think they're less so these days.

I was pretty fat before I started to low carb and lost 56 pounds over the first year and thankfully those pounds have remained lost ever since.

I really love my food, look forward to every meal and still get a thrill out of being as slim as I was in my 20's. I like how easy it can be to follow the principles when eating out too, there always seem to be options on menus almost everywhere. OK, perhaps not Pizza Hut, but hey...

I find the diet easy to follow. I found it quickly became instinctive, the principles are straightforward and only exclude a small number of foods which are themselves inherently unhealthy.

I'm type 1, so I will always be insulin dependent although I use much less insulin than I used to. That in itself is an advantage since blood sugar levels don't fluctuate as wildly as they tended to when following a higher carbohydrate diet. Lower doses equate with less uncertainty over the outcome.

Diane's story

I'm now 30 years old and have had diabetes for 26 years since the age of 4. My current HbA1c is 6.7. Even though it was so long ago, I remember feeling tired, thirsty, very unwell and sick before I was diagnosed.

Before I started low carbing, my diet was not very good. I ate a lot of carbohydrate-laden meals, such as pasta, bread, potatoes, and cereals and did not eat a lot of vegetables and hardly any fruit. I was always tired, bloated and flatulent! I felt heavy, and I had put a lot of weight on over the years with increased insulin needs and the heavy meals I was eating.

The dieticians at the hospital diabetes clinic always advised me to have at least 60% of carbohydrate in every meal, and a low carb diet was never discussed. Eventually news about the success of other diabetics on a low carb approach to diet filtered through and as I wanted to lose weight I decided to attend Dr Morrison.

I have been trying to stick to this method for two years or so now. It hasn't always run smoothly. I have fallen on and off the low carb wagon! However, I have been actively following and enjoying a low-carbohydrate diet for a number of months now with no slip ups.

I eat between 50-100g of carbohydrate per day, and this is mainly made up of fruit-based carb. My typical breakfast is a chopped banana with natural yoghurt, mixed nuts, a sprinkle of cinnamon and crumbled oatcakes. Sometimes I will have a frozen fruit and natural yoghurt smoothie with cinnamon. Snack is a chopped apple and carrot with feta cheese or rice cakes with sugar-free peanut butter. Lunch is protein (chicken, lamb or eggs) with a salad with olive oil and mixed seeds. Dinner is meat with vegetables and if a curry, I have a small amount of basmati rice or quinoa. On occasion, I have a portion of sweet potato with dinner. If I have a dessert, it's usually a banana mashed with sugar-free peanut butter. Throughout the day I drink a lot of green tea. I have also replaced cow's milk with almond and soya milk.

I do miss pasta on occasion, and I miss crisps, although I have replaced these with baked crispy curly kale.

When I am following a low-carbohydrate diet I have a lot more energy, am not as bloated, and my digestion is far better. My blood sugars are stable, and this alone makes me feel happy.

Aside from my blood sugars being better, my skin is a lot clearer, and I have the energy to walk longer.

I have not lost a lot of weight, but rather have inches. I love the variety of interesting and tasty foods I eat, discovering new foods and feeling fine and satisfied after a meal, instead of heavy and bloated.

The diet is easy to follow. Once you go through the first 14 days, you no longer miss caffeine and appreciate the lighter feeling of fullness you have.

I take metformin as I have "double diabetes" and use insulin.

CHAPTER 5

MANAGING YOUR MEDICATIONS AS YOU CUT YOUR CARBOHYDRATES

You will have seen in the previous chapters just how counterproductive at best, and just plain dangerous at worst, a high carb/low fat/low protein diet is for diabetics of all types.

If you had previously been eating the sorts of food recommended by various governments as "healthy for everyone" you will now be intending to:

1. Upping your protein at each meal. In some cases, you will be doubling the amount you eat

2. Cutting back on refined carbohydrates a great deal

3. Eating more non-starchy vegetables

4. Eating the same or less sweet fruit

5. Cutting back on processed foods, such as crisps, commercial sauces, biscuits and sweets

6. Cutting back severely on processed seed and vegetable oils

7. Adding back mono-unsaturated fat (such as olive oil) and naturally saturated animal fat to add necessary calories if you are already slim to replace the calories lost from refined carbohydrate

8. Adding back only enough mono-unsaturated fat and naturally saturated animal fat needed for cooking and for adding to food to make it taste good if you have weight to lose.

Insulin users should be aiming for three meals a day, say at 8am, 1pm and 6pm to prevent insulin stacking. This timing allows for at least enough time for the previous insulin dose used to cover the meal to 'clear' before the next meal. If such meal times don't suit you, try to have at least five hours between main meals[66].

Non-insulin users can be more flexible about their meals, and you may choose to have several small meals a day if this suits you better.

Let us now review what types of insulin work best for different circumstances.

Here is a review of the insulins that are currently available in the UK[67].

RAPID ACTING INSULINS FOR SUGARY/STARCHY CARB AND CORRECTION DOSES:

These start to work in 15 minutes, peak at just over one hour, are almost done by three hours and have a tail of five hours.

1. Aspart also known as NovoRapid pen fill cartridges for Novopen or disposable Flexpen or disposable Flextouch

2. Lispro also known as Humalog in cartridge for Autopen Classic or Humapen or the disposable Humalog Kwikpen

3. Glulisine also known as Apidra cartridge for ClikSTAR or Autopen 24 and disposable in Solostar.

REGULAR ACTING INSULIN FOR LOW STARCH VEGETABLES, PROTEIN AND FATTY/MEATY MEALS:

These start to work in 45 minutes, peak at 2.5 hours, mainly gone by five hours and with a tail of up to eight hours.

1. Hypurin Porcine Neutral for Autopen Classic

2. Actrapid vial for injection with syringe and needle

3. Humulin S Autopen Classic or Humapen

4. Insuman Rapid for ClikSTAR and Autopen 24

LONG ACTING INSULIN FOR DAY AND NIGHT TIME COVER

These insulins start to work in 1-2 hours, peak at 4-12 hours and last 16-42 hours.

1. Insulin Degludec also known as Tresiba pen fill cartridges or in Flextouch disposable pen

2. Insulin Detemir also known as Levemir comes in cartridges for Novopens or Flexpen disposable or Levemir Innolet. This is given twice a day

3. Insulin Glargine also known as Lantus available in cartridges for the ClikSTAR or Autopen 24 or from the disposable Lantus Solostar. This insulin is suitable for once daily administration

4. Insulin Glargine via the Toujeo using the Solostar pen is three times as concentrated as Lantus

5. Hypurin Bovine Lente vial and syringe only

6. Hypurin Bovine Isophane cartridges for Autopen and Classic

7. Hypurin Porcine Isophane cartridges for Autopen and Classic

8. Insulatard via Penfill for Novopens or Insulatard Innolet

9. Humulin I via cartridges for Autopen Classic or Humapen or disposable Humulin I Kwikpen

10. Insuman Basal via cartridge for ClikSTAR or Autopen 24 or Insuman Basal Solostar.

MIXED INSULINS OR BIPHASIC INSULINS

These are mixed insulins in the same cartridge, and the aim is to provide a basal insulin with some meal support with breakfast and the evening meal. They are mainly used for type 2 diabetes but were commonly used in type 1s up to eight years ago, especially on newly-diagnosed diabetics in the UK.

1. Novomix 30 (30% fast acting) via Penfill cartridges for Novopens or in a disposable Flexpen.

2. Humalog mix 25 (25% fast acting) for cartridges for Autopen Classic or Humapen or Kwikpen.

3. Humalog mix 50 (50% fast acting) for cartridges for Autopen Classic or Humapen or Kwikpen.

4. Hypurin Porcine 30/70 mix. (30% fast acting) cartridges for Autopen Classic.

5. Humulin M3 (30% fast acting) cartridges for Autopen Classic or Humapen or Kwikpen.

6. Insuman Comb 15 (15% fast acting) cartridge for Autopen 24 or ClikSTAR.

7. Insuman Comb 25 (25% fast acting) cartridge for Autopen 24 or ClikSTAR.

8. Insuman Comb 50 (50% fast acting) cartridge for Autopen 24 or ClikSTAR.

Necessary changes you need to make to insulin for type ones on a basal/bolus regime:

Changes to monitoring

Whatever monitoring schedule you have been on, you will probably need to increase the frequency of blood tests over the carbohydrate reduction period.

You will need a minimum of five test strips a day and more if you exercise or drive.

Take your blood sugar:

1. On waking

2. Before lunch

3. Before dinner

4. Before bed

5. At 2-4am once or twice a week till your basal insulin has become stable.

6. Before exercising.

7. After exercising.

8. One hour after stopping exercising.

9. If you feel low at any time.

10. Before driving. (Your blood sugar must be over 5.0 to drive!)

11. After each hour of driving.

12. If you feel unwell.

13. During periods of illness, e.g. the cold or flu or gastroenteritis check every 2.5 - 5 hours and act on the results, including during the night.

Ouch! My poor fingers...

Ah yes, your fingers may well soon resemble pin cushions...

Modern lancets and blood-pricking devices are relatively gentle and, when you are testing on such a regular basis, you will quickly get used to them. It's wise to move around the fingers of each hand to ensure one particular area doesn't get targeted all the time. I must admit, I use the fingers on my right hand more than the left because I'm left-handed and I don't want my dominant hand leaking blood on everything, but I do move around the fingers.

Aim for the area clear of the nail to stop the blood seeping behind your nails (it's difficult to clean). It also helps if you gently squeeze the tip of the finger a few times before pricking to encourage blood flow.

Insulin that initially stays the same:

Basal insulin will usually stay the same if you are perfectly matched with it.

You will need less GRADUALLY as you become less insulin resistant and you start to lose weight. This is the main reason for periodic checking of the 2-4am blood sugar.

I suggest that every time you lose seven pounds or more in weight that you do some 2-4am blood sugars to check that your basal level is still correct for you. If you see low blood sugars of less than 5.0 overnight, you need to cut your basal insulin.

The morning blood sugar is not completely reliable for checking basal insulin levels because in about half of all adult diabetics and almost all adolescent diabetics the dawn phenomenon raises the morning level. The hormone cortisol is released from your adrenal glands midway through the night. Its job is to gear up the body for the day. It also counteracts the effects of insulin making you more insulin resistant[68].

Unless you have an insulin pump, there is a limited amount you can do about the dawn phenomenon. You can give 2/3 of your total basal dose at bedtime and the other third in the morning to see if that works, but you must make sure your 2-4am blood sugars are not too low. If this is not working out for you, you really just need to give yourself a correction dose of rapid acting insulin when you wake up. The main thing is to adjust your basal insulin according to the 2-4am level and not the blood sugar you check first thing in the morning so that you don't end up giving yourself too much basal insulin at night and inadvertently ending up with a hypo during the night.

Many type 1s take more basal than they really need because they are relying on it to cover some of the carbohydrates from their starchy meals. If you are doing this, then you will need to cut basal insulin quite sharply after you start a restricted carbohydrate diet.

Insulin to add:

When you are cutting your carbohydrates, the focus of your new meal plan should be on protein and low starch vegetables rather than starch. As a result, you can no longer just ignore the protein component of your meal which in most cases will be 3-8oz (75-225g) in size for each meal.

Few diabetics have been supplied with insulin that is suitable to cover protein. It is easiest to use older insulins called "regular" insulin. In days of old, these used to be the only insulin apart from long acting basal insulin that was available. For many years they were the only insulins to cover meals. They have now been largely replaced by the rapid acting insulins such as Humalog, NovoRapid and Apidra.

These rapid-acting insulins are much better at covering refined carbohydrate than the regular insulins or for giving correction doses when you want to lower a high blood sugar.

However, there is a worthwhile place for the old regular insulins as they last 5-8 hours and are perfect for covering protein[69] , non-starchy vegetables and meals with a lot of meat, pasta and fat such as pizza, lasagne, pasta with creamy/meaty sauces and moussaka.

Humulin S and Insuman Rapid are "human insulin" and Hypurin Neutral which is the pork insulin are all available in cartridge form for pens. Actrapid is available in vials for use with needles and syringes. Pump users will use an extended bolus to cover protein.

The formula for covering protein is 2 units of regular insulin for every deck of cards size of meat or portion of around 3oz[70] (75g) . You will need correspondingly more if you are insulin resistant.

The highest amount of insulin you will inject in any one shot will be seven units. This is so that the insulin gets absorbed rapidly and evenly by the tissues and does not hang about. By this method, pioneered by diabetologists Dr John Bantle and then by Dr Richard Bernstein[71], you will find that your pens act with the same degree of efficiency as insulin pumps.

For a person with low insulin resistance, an average portion of meat 6-7oz (150-175g) will need about seven units to cover it given as a single shot.

A large steak will take about 10 hours to fully digest. Therefore, it is better to give half the estimated insulin with the meal and leave the remainder for another injection three hours after starting the meal.

Lasagne and moussaka can be made low-carb by substituting sliced courgette for the pasta sheets in the lasagne and omitting the potato and just using aubergine in moussaka. These can then be covered by regular insulin, usually in a single dose.

Pasta dishes can be simulated by using courgette or squash for the pasta strips. You may need a spiral vegetable cutter for this. If you think you miss pasta, maybe it's just the delicious sauces that have been created for the dishes and almost any pasta sauce will go well a plain chicken breast. This would be then covered with regular insulin in one shot. Cheese sauce can be made with double cream, grated cheese and seasoning. You don't need any flour at all with this substitution. If you are eating the pasta and potato versions of lasagne and moussaka, you will probably need to split the insulin and give some with the meal and the remainder about three hours after starting to eat.

Fish and shellfish are quickly digested and are usually covered in a single shot of regular insulin.

Pizza is particularly hard to cover well. Unlike the other dishes, the starch cannot be omitted or de-emphasized to any great extent. There are substitute pizza bases, but they are rarely of the same consistency as "normal" pizza.

Pizza takes eight hours to digest. Like steak or other heavy meat dishes, you will need to space apart the regular insulin injections to cover it. The formula is one unit of regular insulin for every 8g of carbohydrate in the pizza if you have no insulin resistance problems.

You can see that if a meat dish or pizza take 8-10 hours to digest, they will still be raising blood sugars and the insulin needed to cover them will still be active by the time your next meal is due. They could also interfere with your 2-4am blood sugars on which you are calculating your basal insulin levels if you eat them at dinner time.

THE PROBLEMS WITH PIZZA

By experimentation, we have found that it becomes impossible to accurately cover 90g of carbohydrate in any meal and for that reason, pizza slices should be recommended, rather than eating a whole one by yourself which will cause blood sugar chaos...

The most pizza to eat at one time is three slices of regular pizza, and even then it could play havoc with your blood sugars. If you are insulin resistant, the problem could be worse. If you are dining out with friends either order something else or only eat one or two slices, but eat the topping from the rest of the pizza. You are then eating 30-60g carbohydrate, and this is much more manageable.

Insulin to cut:

Basal insulin may need to be cut, but this is usually a gradual process. Nevertheless, in the first week, check the 2-4am blood sugars every 3 days to make sure that it is above 5.0. (US 90).

The rapid acting insulin that you have been using to cover all components of your meals will be correspondingly reduced as you cut the carbohydrate component for your meals.[72]

There are several ways of going about making the changes to your regime.

Recommended method for insulin users: Gradual reduction one meal at a time.

1. Learn to count carbohydrates.

The online course at D-solve.com has a section on this, as has the very good B-DEC online course.

The book, Carbs and Cals, Protein and Fat, by Chris Cheyette and Yello Balolia, shows pictures of food in different portion sizes to guide you. There is also a phone app with the same information. These can be found on Amazon in both the UK and US.

The Collins Gem Carbohydrate counting book is excellent. CalorieKing is a beneficial website. It is US based.

The USDA site has many carbohydrate indexes listed for different foods. You then simply need to weigh the food to find its carb count.

Nutritional scales can be bought for about £30, sometimes more, sometimes less. These are helpful to use in the house, but when Dr Morrison and her son were learning to eyeball portions, they took it with them to restaurants so they could weigh things. This gets you outstanding service because the restaurant thinks you are food inspectors!

Paradoxically, the tighter your carb control in the diet, the less you need to carb count. This is because the average carb count of low starch vegetables is about 5g of carbohydrate.

If you eat larger portions of refined carbohydrate in baked goods, rice and so forth, it becomes essential to get your carb counting skills consistent and precise, because you are basing your insulin injections on your sums.

2. Start using the 7-unit rule for all your insulin injections.

This will make all of your insulin more efficient, so cut your basal and meal insulin by 20% from the very start. This means that you will be giving multiple injections at least to start with. Once you have cut your carbohydrates in your meals, however, you probably won't need more than two injections for each meal.

3. Up the protein in your meals and start covering it with regular insulin.

Remember the formula, 2 units regular insulin for every 3oz (75g) or card deck size of meat. Again, this is a maximum of 7 units per shot. Use multiple shots if necessary and space them appropriately if you are eating a large steak or pizza.

4. Stop snacking between meals.

This can be harder than it sounds. Snacking seems to be an ingrained habit for many. Eating from the communal biscuit tin appears to be common in many workplaces. It can be an effort to stop eating something with tea or coffee at break times.

The increased protein and the decreased snacking go hand in hand. You should be peckish, but not ravenous when it comes to your next meal. If you are hungry, is your blood sugar too low before your meal? You may need to cut your rapid insulin that you have been giving at your previous meal.

Sometimes the snacks have been covered to some extent by basal insulin levels that are really too high. You may need to cut basal doses too. Unexplained hypos during the day are a sign that your morning basal doses are too high.

Night basals are adjusted by paying attention to the 2-4am blood sugars. If you have been in the habit of having a bedtime snack and you stop this, you may need to cut your night basal if this has been covering it.

5. Cut carbs and insulin one meal at a time

Cut your breakfast carbohydrate in half. Cut your breakfast rapid insulin in half too.

After a few days of checking blood sugars and adjusting your insulin for that meal, you should be having pre-lunch blood sugars of 4-7.

Now cut your breakfast carbohydrate to no more than 30g. This is the level at which most people can still have linear matching of insulin to carbohydrate. Adjust your insulin level so that your pre-lunch blood sugars are 4-7 and you do not need any snacks for low blood sugars.

You will find that you need a certain amount of rapid acting insulin to cover 30g of carbohydrate.

Once breakfast is stable, you can start to work on cutting your lunch carbohydrate in exactly the same way. First cut the carb and insulin in half and then adjust till you are having no snacks, no hypos and blood sugars of 4-7 before dinner. Then cut to 30g of carbohydrate and adjust as before. You will usually find that you need less insulin to cover this amount of carbohydrate compared to breakfast.

The advantage of cutting down one meal at a time is that you need focus your extra blood sugar monitoring on one part of the day rather than the whole lot at once. It also gets you used to different sorts of food at various meals.

Most breakfasts tend to be egg based when you start low carbing. It helps to experiment with low carb baking as this can taste even better than regular wheat/cereal based breakfasts and does you good instead of harm. Because low carb baking is usually nut and whey-protein based, it fills you up for longer, and you don't feel hungry between meals. The dishes also usually freeze well and don't go mouldy as quickly as wheat based goods.

Lunch tends to be based around different soups, cold meats and salads. If you make enough for meals at night, such as roasting two chickens instead of one, you can have enough leftovers for lunches.

The next meal to get right is the evening meal. Again, try cutting the carbohydrates in half and then cutting to 30g maximum in a two-stage process.

For many people who eat a traditional meal with meat, potatoes and vegetables, the only changes are to up the meat portion a bit, cut the starch element, and add more vegetables, preferably the low-starch type. They can have the pleasure of adding butter to vegetables to improve their taste. For people who tend to have pizza or pasta based meals, or meals based around rice, there can be more adjustment to be made.

6. Learn your insulin sensitivity at different times of the day

Most people find that for 30g of carbohydrate they need the most insulin at breakfast, the next highest amount at dinner time and the least at lunch. This reflects your carbohydrate sensitivity for that time of day. How many grams of carbohydrate can you eat for one unit of insulin? This number is important. You can use it to cover different sizes of carbohydrate meals in the future so you can be more flexible with your meals.

For the time being, I am trying to get you used to eating 30g of carb three times a day, eating enough protein, avoid snacking, and getting your basals tuned in. The main issue is to prevent serious hypoglycaemia. During this phase while you are working out your insulin sensitivity, it is best to avoid strenuous or prolonged exercise as this adds another factor into an already unstable situation.

Women: learn your insulin sensitivity after your period is over.

Women will find that they are best to start the programme soon after their period has finished. Figuring out new basal levels and meal insulin sensitivity will be necessary for the run up to and during the period, but this adds too much complexity at this stage.

Once you get healthy blood sugars in your best two weeks, you can get to grips with your hormonal challenges at other phases of your menstrual cycle.

These difficulties will not be necessarily applicable to women who are on methods of contraception that produce no periods or who are stable hormonally. This topic is discussed further in the FAQ section of this book.

Methods that can be used for type 2s:

Gradual reduction of carbohydrate across all meals till you are at 30g for each meal three times a day.

This is good for the carb-addicted who may get real withdrawals from missing their favourite hit. This method is perfect for those who do not use insulin or oral hypoglycaemic drugs. You will see improvements fast.

Those using sulphonylureas and glinides will need to monitor blood sugars and cut their doses or even omit them entirely. More advice is given on this in the drugs section.

For insulin users this method is doable, but requires vigilance across the whole day, and at least once at night. It is, therefore, better to stick to the recommended method if you can. If you mainly want to cut down carbs by this method and have a week's holiday, can stop driving, and have family support to help you, then this option may suit you. It is best to cut your insulin doses before you cut your carbs.

Cold Turkey to 30g across all meals.

This method can be used by all types of diabetics but is most suitable for those who are not using insulin or oral hypoglycaemics.

Ideally, they should already be good cooks/bakers and have good family support.

Insulin users and oral hypoglycaemic drug users are best to cut their doses by one-third or even one-half and then adjust the dose up or down depending on the response to this method.

It is the fastest way to get blood sugars in gear, but it is the riskiest method for hypoglycaemia. Is there any particular reason why you need to do it this way?

Cold Turkey to 30g one meal at a time.

This is faster than the gradual method and can be a good compromise for those insulin /oral hypoglycaemic users who want to see immediate results on their blood sugars.

Again, the plan would be to cut that meal's insulin dose by 1/3 to ½ and then adjust the insulin up or down. Ideally, start at the beginning of the day. This gives you all day when you are usually awake to measure blood sugars more frequently and adjust doses of medication.

All cold turkey methods are not suitable if you are driving that day. These methods are more easily done when you are on holiday, off at the weekend and particularly when you are not going to be in the house alone. Family members should know what you are doing, why you are doing it, and know to treat hypoglycaemia.

Necessary changes for type 2s on insulin

Type twos on insulin need to go through the same process as for type ones. Within quite a short period of time, they will generally go one of three routes. The route will depend on how low they consistently cut their carbs and how much beta cell activity they have left.

They still need basal insulin, regular insulin and rapid acting insulin, the same as type ones. Their pancreas cannot cope without a high degree of insulin support. Their doses may be reduced from previously, but they cannot stop insulin or pancreatic support drugs.

They don't need any meal insulin at all and just need to keep their basal insulin going. In this case, their pancreas can cope with the lighter carb load.

They find that they don't need any insulin anymore at all.

Type twos who are able to come off insulin and have normal blood sugars often feel that they have been cured. They are actually in remission and need to be vigilant about their diet lifelong.

Type 2s who use biphasic insulins

Biphasic insulins often work well with a low-carb diet. There is, however, almost no way that you can alter your insulin dose to fit the meal.

You will be giving yourself your usual doses of insulin, and by recording your blood sugar response to meals, you can see where you need more insulin and when you need less. You can then see your doctor to see if you would prefer to alter the carbohydrate you are eating at various meals to accommodate the insulin you are on, change to a different biphasic insulin, or switch to a purely basal insulin or change to separate insulins for basal and for meal coverage.

Should you prefer to stay with a biphasic insulin, you will see that you will have some insulin coverage for carbohydrate at breakfast and with your evening meal but almost none with your lunch. The dawn phenomenon is active at breakfast and means that the same dose of insulin at this time will not be as effective as that injected at dinner time.

The main thing that is useful is to allocate your total daily carbohydrate to where there is enough injected insulin/pancreatic function to cover it. A way of doing this instead of 30g carb at each meal is to eat say, 30g of carbohydrate at breakfast, 15g of carbohydrate for lunch, and 45g carbohydrate at your evening meal.

If you prefer more carbohydrate at lunch than is adequately covered by biphasic insulin, you may need to inject a rapid-acting insulin to cover it at lunch time. This means three injections a day minimum, but this is still fewer injections than in a basal-bolus regime.

Necessary changes to type 2s on oral hypoglycaemic drugs

The first thing to establish is, are you on any of these drugs?[73] What are the drugs that can lower blood sugars? Those that act primarily on post meal blood sugars.

Sulphonylureas

This group of drugs have the strongest effect on the pancreas when it comes to making the pancreas secrete insulin. They are likely to need to be reduced as you cut carbohydrate. The extent to which this needs to be done must be individualised by monitoring your blood sugars.

1. Glibenclamide 5mg to 15mg daily

2. Gliclazide 40-320mg daily also known as Diamicron and both are available in the long acting M/R versions

3. Glimepiride 1mg-6mg daily also known as Amaryl

4. Glipizide 2.5-20mg daily also known as Minodiab

5. Tolbutamide 0.5-1.5mg daily.

Glinides

This group of drugs are similar to sulphonylureas, but they have a much narrower time of action. They are likely to need to be reduced as you cut carbohydrate. The extent to which this needs to be done must be individualised by monitoring your blood sugars.

Nateglinide 60mg three times a day also known as Starlix.

Repaglinide 500micrograms up to four times a day with each main meal up to 4mg with each dose.

Gliptans

These drugs make the pancreas secrete insulin when you eat, but also suppress glucagon and reduce gastric emptying. They produce fewer hypoglycaemia episodes than the sulphonylureas or the glinides, but again you will need to monitor blood sugar levels. It may be that you won't need to take these drugs when your carb intake is reduced enough.

1. Sitagliptan also known as Januvia in 25mg, 50mg and 100mg once daily.

2. Linagliptan also known as Trajenta 5mg once daily.

3. Saxagliptan also known as Onglyza 2.5 or 5mg once daily.

4. Vidagliptan also known as Galvus is 50mg twice daily.

FLOZINs

Dapagliflozin 5mg and 10mg, Canagliflozin 100mg and 300mg, and Empagliflozin 10mg and 25mg work on the kidney to increase glucose excretion and reduce glucose reabsorption. As they do have a mechanism for reducing blood glucose, it is best to check your blood sugar over the transition period. They also help people lose weight and lower the blood pressure. They have a small chance of causing ketoacidosis in type two diabetics even when the blood sugars are not raised very much.

Injectables for type 2s.

The main benefit of these drugs is that they often improve weight loss in type two diabetics. One of their actions is to increase secretion of insulin so blood sugars should be monitored if you are transitioning to a low carb diet.

1. Exanitide also known as Byetta 5 or 10 units twice a day.

2. Liraglutide also known as Victoza, start at 0.6 units then up to 1.2 and possibly 1.8 once daily.

3. Lixisenatide also known as Lyxumia 10units or 20units once daily.

Acarbose is a drug that reduces the absorption of sucrose from the diet. It is not used that much because of its gastric side effects. If you are taking this in conjunction with a low carb diet, you may as well stop the drug. You won't have to monitor blood sugars unless you are also on one of the other drugs previously mentioned or insulin.

Those that reduce insulin resistance

Metformin 500mg-2g daily. Also known as Glucophage. Available in M/R forms that cause less diarrhoea. You don't need to monitor blood sugars on this drug unless you are also on one of the drugs that do reduce blood sugar or insulin. You may need to cut this medication in dose or perhaps stop completely if you normalise your weight. It is worth getting your HbA1c tested every time you drop half a stone to see if you need to cut the dose.

Glitazones

Pioglitazone is the only drug in this category at present in the UK. Rosiglitazone is also licenced in the USA. Both drugs reduce insulin resistance. You don't need to monitor blood sugars on this medication unless you are also on one of the drugs that do reduce blood sugar or insulin. You may need to cut this drug in dose or perhaps stop completely if you normalise your weight. It is worth getting your HbA1c tested every time you drop half a stone to see if you need to cut the dose.

How do you adjust them?

For drugs that reduce insulin resistance, I suggest getting an HbA1c check every half stone weight loss till your weight or blood sugars are normalized on a low carb diet. This means 30g or less for each meal. This way your doctor can see if you need any dose adjustment to your drugs.

Users of drugs and insulin that have a direct effect on lowering blood sugar need to be monitored more precisely. Insulin users will be doing blood tests as advised which is to test five or more times a day.

Users of hypoglycaemic drugs need only do this level of monitoring over the period of transition. If this is you, once stable, you can omit blood sugar tests and only need to recheck at half-stone intervals on your way to your ideal weight.

Driving

Drivers need to remember that if they are on insulin, they always have to check their blood sugar before setting off and at one hourly intervals. They must have a blood sugar over 5.0[74].

They must have fast acting carbohydrate to use if their blood sugar is less than 5.0 and preferably glucose in drink, tablet or gel form in the car that they will use if their blood sugars drop below 4.0. They must wait, preferably 30-45 minutes, till their blood sugars, vision, awareness and response times are normal. While they are recovering, even if they feel fine, they are best to take the keys out of the ignition and sit in another seat other than the driver's seat.

Users of hypoglycaemic drugs need to take the same precautions when driving as insulin users when they are transitioning on to a lower carb diet and cutting their medications. Once they are completely stable regarding weight, carbohydrate, blood sugars and medication, they can be more relaxed.

Overnight

Insulin users are best to have company overnight over the period of transition. To avoid night hypoglycaemia, I recommend the steps in the "recommended method".

Cutting the insulin by 20% at the adoption of the 7 unit rule, cutting the insulin again by ½ to 1/3 before cutting a meal to 30g of carb are methods that should give you protection against severe hypoglycaemia.

You will, of course, need to check blood sugars vigilantly and be consistent with your diet. You may need to correct insulin doses up or down depending on response.

Drugs that do NOT affect blood sugars but that may need to be adjusted downwards.

Blood pressure drugs

Low carb dieting often results in a normalisation of blood pressure. This happens because less insulin is being secreted or needed and your weight normalises too.

You may be eating a lot less salt that has previously been hidden in bread and processed foods, and you will retain less fluid due to the lesser amount of glycogen in the muscles and liver. You will tend to excrete more sodium as well. You may need a reduction in the number of medications you take for blood pressure or the doses.

Remember to get your BP done standing up. Get it checked every half stone you lose.

Statins

Statins are now prescribed to nearly every type 2 diabetic and all type 1s over the age of 40 or who have developed any complications.

If they are being used for primary prevention, you don't have any complications from diabetes, and you reach normal blood sugars and are confident you can stick to low carbing for the foreseeable future, then the question is why take them?

These drugs can worsen insulin resistance and have side effects affecting about 10% of those who take them. My point of view is that if you render yourself metabolically normal through low carb dieting, proper insulin management and exercise and you have turned yourself into what I call a "super-diabetic" you have then ceased to have the same reduced life expectancy and morbidity of your less fortunate fellow diabetics. You can re-think all the doom and gloom stuff. You do, of course, have to keep up vigilance and your good habits.

Orlistat

This is the only drug left at present for weight control in the UK, although a few more may be released soon. It works by preventing some of the fat that you eat being absorbed by the gut. Obviously, there are two good reasons why you should stop this drug if you are cutting your carbs. Firstly, this medication is only meant to be used with low-fat diets, which your new diet is not. Secondly, you will have horrendous diarrhoea if you continue to take it with a higher fat diet.

If you are achieving good weight loss with this drug on a low-fat diet, you may be best to continue with it until you have reached your goal weight. You can see how your blood sugars are doing at that point and consider whether to switch diet or not.

If you are not losing weight with Orlistat and particularly if your blood sugars are too high, you may be best to switch now.

Drugs that do NOT affect blood sugars, but that may need to be adjusted upwards.

Painkilling drugs for legs

If you are getting treatment for neuropathy, you can experience a worsening of the pain as your blood sugars come under control. This does resolve over a period of months, but you may need a temporary increase in pain medications.

Nerve damage heals at only about one inch a month. The taller you are, the longer it takes to improve and reverse neuropathy. Foot ulcers are due to a mixture of factors. The improvement in blood sugars can result in much faster resolution of the ulcers.

Other issues that change on a low carb diet

Eye checks

If you have very rapid improvement in your blood sugar, it can lead to shrinkage of swollen endothelial cells and an increased chance of leakage or bleeding from proliferative retinopathy in your eyes. This does not occur if you don't have proliferative retinopathy.

If you DO have proliferative retinopathy, try the gradual reduction in dietary carbohydrate so that your blood sugars also reduce more gradually. Also, you should not take part in any jarring exercise, for example running, trampolining, or activities that increase venous pressure in the head such as headstands or other inverted yoga postures. It is better that you get your blood sugars gradually under control, say over six months, than get them under control in one to two weeks which can be expected with this programme.

Meal planning

So that you don't just pick any old thing off the supermarket shelves here are some ideas... Write down the ingredients you will need to make four main meals over the week. You can get ideas from this book, other cook books and web sites. Carry this list with you when you shop. Look at the discounted food items. Are they suitable for meals? If so get them. If not, stick to your list or some of it. Cook generous portions so that you have leftovers, and bacon and eggs, omelettes and other simple meals can keep you going till the next main shop.

Shopping

You are going to be relying on fresh food that can spoil quickly. Instead of a single large weekly shop, you are likely to need to shop about two or three times a week.

If you get your fresh food once a week, eat the seafood items fastest, and then eat by out of date order the meats that will go out of date the fastest. By the end of the week, you may need to buy fresh ingredients for a further one or two meals before the next big shop.

Cooking

Meal arrangement, which is fine when you start off, consists of putting together single items such as meats, vegetables, fruits and cheeses to make a meal.

Many of us have stopped cooking family meals and have come to rely on take-out meals and processed food. These are often loaded with carbohydrate to bulk them out. This sort of food is not good for you, so the sooner you learn to make a few good, hearty meals that you can produce a few times a month, the better. We have some recipes later in the book and also give book and website recommendations in the appendices, and we promise you that low-carbohydrate cooking need not be either time-consuming or difficult.

Baking

To really make the most of your new low carb diet, learn to bake the low carb way. Your breakfasts can move away from eggs with everything, and you can find good substitutes for many items that you may otherwise miss.

Next Steps

This chapter has focused on the main stages that insulin users and those using oral hypoglycaemic drugs need to take to transition safely from a high carb diet to a low carb diet.

You will be able to eat 30g of carb with each meal. This is a moderate amount of carb to eat on a low carb diet. Some of you will want to go lower and get even better blood sugar control or freedom from injected insulin/medications. Some of you may be planning a pregnancy, or you may want to reverse complications of diabetes. Some of you would like to be able to eat more than 30g of carb with each meal.

The next chapter will look at what blood sugar levels and carb levels are suitable for the needs of various people at different ages and stages of their life, and discuss what you need to know if you want to eat lower or higher amounts of carbs than 30g for three main meals a day.

CHAPTER SUMMARY

This chapter gives you a lot of information to take in, and you will probably need to read over the sections that apply to you several times before it starts to make sense, but here is a basic sum-up:

1. We recommend you start by cutting carbs to 30g for each meal to work out how to make your medications match what you need.

2. When you start low-carb eating, ensure your family knows and is supportive. It's best not to drive or exercise while you start on the programme.

3. The rules are different for insulin users and non-insulin users. Insulin users need to work out their insulin sensitivity and should work towards the gradual reduction of carbohydrates, whereas people not using insulin or oral hypoglycaemic drugs can move to low carbohydrates more quickly if this is what they want to do.

4. You will need to learn to count carbohydrates.

5. You will need to plan your meals and your shopping.

6. You may experience rapid improvements in blood sugar control and how you feel.

CHAPTER 6

PLANNING AND ACHIEVING BLOOD SUGAR TARGETS

The next two chapters go into detail about managing your medication and describe the different daily carbohydrate totals you should aim for, depending on your goals and/or any existing diabetic complications.

Eating 30g of carbohydrate three times a day, using the methods described, should put most diabetics of both type one and two into the range of 5.5-6.5 for their HbA1c. Some people may experience higher HbA1c levels, particularly if they have any features of metabolic syndrome[75]. This may lessen as they continue to lose weight.

Dr Jorgen Neilsen has achieved average HbA1cs of 6.4% for type ones and 5.8% for type twos patients on 70-90g of carb a day[76] , and Dr Lois Jovanovich gets her pregnant patients to HbA1cs well under 6.0 % on 30g-45g of carb three or four times a day[77] . (Pregnant women can be ravenous).

A big plus of a low carb diet is that once your carbohydrate intakes and insulin doses are stabilised, severe hypoglycaemia episodes happen a lot less than with regular diets and your blood sugar fluctuations are far less. This can be great if you drive a lot or you are planning a pregnancy.

How to use blood sugar targets

The blood sugar goals we have given in the boxes are approximate values based on those given by the American Diabetes Society and the International Diabetes Federation[78]. It has been increasingly recognised that post meal blood sugars have a lot more influence on the long-term blood sugar value of your HbA1c than the overnight fasting blood sugar levels[79]. This is helpful to know because striving for "perfect" first thing blood sugars can put you at risk of low blood sugars overnight.

This is not only dangerous but is counter-productive because of the high blood sugars that can result from over treating hypos and also the adrenaline system coming into action and causing a flood of glucose to be released from the liver. For those of you who are affected by the dawn phenomenon, you may not be able to escape high blood sugars first thing, even when the 2-4am blood sugars are in the 4-6mmol/l range.

A recent study showed that you can "get away with" morning blood sugars quite a bit higher than post meal blood sugars. This is a good thing because post meal blood sugars are a lot easier to control with simple dietary manipulation and exercise while early morning blood sugar levels can be particularly stubborn.

For everyone, except pregnant women who have lower blood sugar targets, once your blood sugar is under 4.0mmol you should raise your blood sugar to at least that level. When you anticipate driving, you will need to increase it to 5.0 as a minimum. Everyone can have low blood sugars sporadically, especially since carb counting, glucose release from food, insulin absorption and energy expended on exercise can be variable despite your best efforts.

If you are getting low blood sugars more than very infrequently, then you need to look carefully at factors that could be causing the hypos and adjust your insulin or medications downwards as appropriate. Avoidance of hypoglycaemia is crucial generally, but particularly when you will be alone, or driving and particularly overnight.

The American Diabetes Association actually allows for lower blood sugar targets in certain circumstances. Levels of 3.3mmol are an acceptable lower limit for pregnant women in the first trimester of pregnancy when non-diabetic women have very low blood sugar levels. This relative hypoglycaemia contributes to the nausea of pregnancy.

The low blood-sugar levels are also optimal for healthy foetal development. When seeking to emulate these very low blood sugars pregnant women in the USA may be provided with insulin pumps and subcutaneous blood sugar monitoring systems. They may also receive considerable training in their use[80].

Currently, in the UK, blood sugar management is not as sophisticated as this, and therefore we advise a lower limit of 4.0mmol. Should you be advised that you may go lower to a target between 3.5-3.9mmol by your diabetologist under their strict supervision, then this is fine.

At the other end of the scale, the higher limits we have given, you will need to do one of several things if your average blood sugar for that time of day is over the target value. The most efficient thing is to cut the amount of carbohydrate you eat for the meal eaten before. You can also cut your portion sizes, as long as this does not result in excessive hunger before your next meal. Another idea is to add more fibre to the meal, which can be helpful if you want to lose weight or don't eat as many vegetables as you perhaps should.

You can also add more fat to the meal which is helpful if you are of normal weight or thin. This cuts the blood glucose spike after the meal. You can also take a walk or do another exercise immediately after the given meal. For those on insulin, they also have the option of increasing the insulin to cover that meal.

Who would benefit from tight blood sugar control?

Older children, who accept that some dietary restriction will have long term benefits on their health, are good candidates for the tight blood sugar control that is achievable for most type 1 and type 2 diabetics who eat 30g of carbs three times a day.

Newly diagnosed diabetics, both type 1 and type 2, will put far less stress on their pancreatic beta cells by restricting the carbohydrates in their diet.

Many pregnant women and those planning a pregnancy will "get away" with a dietary intake of 30g of carb per meal.

Experienced insulin pumpers have the extra technology to help them get near normal blood sugars. By cutting to a moderate 30g per meal diet, they can see very good blood sugars, far better than the HbA1cs of 7.3-8.4% averages found in trials of newly diagnosed and experienced type one diabetics using dose adjustment for normal eating (DAFNE).

A recently diagnosed type 1 diabetic who is particularly keen to prolong the honeymoon period as long as possible.

TIGHT BLOOD SUGAR CONTROL

The tight blood sugar control group is defined as:

HbA1c target is 5.5% to 6.5%

8am blood sugar level average 7.0mmol/l

Pre-meals and bedtime blood sugar levels are 4.0-8.0mmol

The one-hour post meal blood sugar level is 9.0mmol.

If you are disappointed at your results some two to three months after stabilising your carb level, then you may wish to consider cutting carbohydrates further to achieve even tighter blood sugar control.

Dr Richard Bernstein advocates a stringent, low-carb diet with 30-42 g of carbohydrate a day: 6g of carb at breakfast because this is the time you are most insulin resistant, 12g for lunch and dinner, with 6g or 12g before bedtime for those who wish this. His patients can get HbA1cs of 4.2-5.4%. The blood sugar fluctuations are minimal with this level of meal to insulin matching.

It is particularly difficult for menstruating women to achieve these lower blood sugar targets, even with rigorous dietary control and exemplary insulin management because of fluctuating hormone levels. Fit, slim, younger men who exercise regularly find it much easier.

Women will still benefit from blood sugar improvement and reduced hypoglycaemia even if they find it very difficult to get an

HbA1c in the 4s. To get to the level of carbohydrates prescribed by Dr Bernstein, the carbohydrate must be nutritious, low starch vegetables and berries, and the Big Bad 8 we referred to in Chapter 2 don't get a look in. Fruit and legumes are also pretty limited.

Who would benefit from extremely tight blood sugar control?

Women who are planning a pregnancy who are happy to go a bit lower on their dietary carbohydrate.

Women who are pregnant and who are not achieving a HbA1c under 6.0 on a 30g per meal moderate low-carb diet or who want to go lower towards non-pregnancy level blood sugars.

Those who have troublesome hypoglycaemia even on 30g per meal moderate low carb diet.

A young adult who has complications of diabetes they wish to reverse.

EXTREMELY TIGHT BLOOD SUGAR CONTROL

The extremely tight blood sugar control group is defined as:

Hba1C target is 4.5% to 5.5%

8am blood sugar level average 6.5mmol/l

Pre-meals and bedtime range blood sugar levels at 4.0-6.0mmol

One hour blood sugar level after starting to eat 8.0mmol

2-6am blood sugar level 4.0-6.0mmol.

Who would be better off with looser control?

Very strict blood sugars are not necessarily the best thing for everyone.

Babies and toddlers have unpredictable eating, sleeping and activity patterns. Insulin is often best given after they have actually eaten. The developing brain is more at risk from recurrent or severe hypoglycaemia. With these difficulties in mind, it is often better to accept a reduction in blood sugar targets and run blood sugars a bit higher.

Once a child is of school age, their eating and activity patterns settle down, and tighter targets can be attempted.

Adolescents have huge hormonal surges that render blood sugars hard to control due to intermittent insulin resistance. There is no problem with type 2s doing strict low carbing should they be willing, but even if they do, blood sugars are not usually as good as for adults over the age of 22.

Type 1 adolescents will also benefit from reduced carb diets, but their blood sugar control will not be as good as for the older age group. Peak insulin resistance is 12-13 for girls and 15-17 for boys. About 3-4 years each side of this, you can expect difficulty in controlling blood sugars, especially the morning blood sugars due to the dawn phenomenon.

Adolescent girls have HbA1cs around 2% higher than boys due to the added effect of menstrual cycles. Those who involve their parents, particularly their mother, in their diabetic care do a lot better than those who choose to go it alone.

Older diabetics, particularly those who have serious comorbidities, have not as much to gain from strict blood sugar control as their younger counterparts. It takes on average, with the poor level of control that goes on in the NHS now, 10-20 years for a diabetic to develop complications that are enough to severely affect their quality of life. For younger diabetics, and particularly children, they have everything to gain from strict blood sugar control, but depending on their life expectancy many older adults may be happy to have looser control.

These blood sugar targets are far tighter than is achieved in the NHS for most type 1s and many type 2s. It should be noted, however, that diabetic complications are accumulating on this level of blood sugar, and even if not apparent right now, trouble is brewing for your future. If you are in the younger age group, try to get back on track when you can and if older, do consider your quality of life as well as any quantity of life.

You will probably be eating 45g of carb for each meal giving you 135g of carbohydrate a day and possibly more.

LOOSER BLOOD SUGAR CONTROL

The loose blood sugar control group is defined as:

Hba1c 7-8%

8am blood sugar average 9mmol

Pre-meal and pre-bed target blood sugar levels – 4.0-10mmol

Post meal one-hour target blood sugar level – 11mmol

Personal variability regarding complications

Although the Diabetes Control and Complications Trial showed an exponential match between higher blood sugars and higher complications, doctors will see patients who are severely affected by complications despite pretty good blood sugars of around HbA1cs of 5.8-7% and others who seem to get away for years with HbA1cs in excess of 9% without apparent difficulty.

Exactly why this happens is not fully known. Obviously, blood sugars are one factor, but there are others that we have not figured out.

It is important that you consider your quality of life and possible life expectancy before you decide to settle for blood sugar targets that may in retrospect be too high for you. Patients sometimes say things like, "I can't give up my bread, potatoes, porridge", or whatever. They may baulk at the time involved in meal preparation and low-carb home baking or indeed the expense of a reduced carbohydrate diet.

For certain types of diabetics, starting at looser control (we like to think of it as Atkins in reverse – you start with a higher number of carbohydrates and shrink the number to suit) makes good sense, and you are better to tighten up on blood sugars gradually.

For some diabetics, blood sugar control can be improved by making daily exercise part of their fitness plan, allowing them to eat more carbohydrate than they otherwise could.

Once you have reached the blood sugar target you have set your mind on, you might always need to think, "Should I actually go lower?"

Who would benefit from "good enough" blood sugar control?

We have discussed the sort of control you are likely to get on 90g of carb a day, who would benefit from going lower to say 40g of carb a day, and who would not actually benefit from trying so hard for normal blood sugars.

There is another group, who may wish to be more gradual in blood sugar reduction or who would prefer to eat more carbohydrate regularly. If you drive a lot, are late middle aged with no complications, are new to an insulin pump or whenever you are switching to a new insulin or delivery method, you may wish to ease up on diabetes control even if this is just temporary.

If you have proliferative retinopathy or peripheral neuropathy and you want to bring your blood sugars down gradually, you may wish to stick with these targets for a few months before going for non-diabetic levels of blood sugar control. You will probably be eating 40g of carb for each meal giving you a daily total of 120g.

"GOOD ENOUGH" BLOOD SUGAR CONTROL

The definition of "good enough" blood sugar control is:

HbA1c range 6-7%

8am blood sugar average 8.0mmol

Pre-meals and bedtime blood sugar levels 4.0-9mmol

Post meal one-hour blood sugar target 10mmol.

How insulin users can eat more or less than 30g of carbohydrates at each meal and still cover it adequately with their insulin:

The previous chapter, which covers the basics of how to get from where you are (what you are eating at the moment) to 30g of carbohydrate for each meal, puts great stress on the fact that everyone who uses insulin should get to this level before they decide on what to do next.

By getting to 30g of carbs for each meal, you will have learned to count carbohydrates – an essential skill for dealing with diabetes – and also learned how much insulin you need to cover these 30g for each meal (if you use insulin). This is your insulin sensitivity, and it can vary widely from person to person.

With this knowledge, you will then be able to vary the carbohydrate in your meals upwards and downwards.

Some of you will want to reduce carbohydrates across the board, and others may want to reduce the amount eaten at certain meals, for example, low-carb breakfasts are relatively easy. Others may want to increase the carbs eaten for certain meals or increase it for all meals.

Reducing carbohydrate in your meals: how to adjust the insulin

Say you need 6 units of rapid-acting insulin to cover 30g of carbohydrate at breakfast, 4 units to cover a 30g lunch, and 5 units to cover a 30g evening meal.

If you wish to cut to 10g carbs at breakfast, 20g at lunch and 25g at dinner, do the sums like this:

1. $30/6$ = one unit of insulin will cover 5g of carb at breakfast. Therefore, to cover 10g of carb at breakfast, you need $10/5$ = 2 units of insulin

2. $30/4$ = one unit of insulin will cover 7.5g of carb at lunch. Therefore, to cover 20g of carb at lunch, you will need $20/7.5$ = 2.6 units of insulin.

Half unit increment pens

You can either inject 3 units of insulin if your pen comes in one-unit increments or you can be more precise by injecting 2.5 units using some of the half-unit pens. Novo Nordisk has demi pens, Novopen junior pens and the echo pens. You will need to switch to NovoRapid from what you are using to use these. Of these, the echo pen is the best of the bunch because it records the amount of insulin you gave at your last shot.

$30/5$= one unit of insulin will cover 6g of carb at your evening meal. Therefore, to cover 25g of carb at dinner you need $25/6$ = 4.16 units of insulin. Just give 4 units of insulin.

For most people, this method will work well. If you have a lot of insulin resistance, you may find you need far less insulin proportionately to cover say 10g than 30g of carbohydrate. You should be able to pick up any alterations you need to make by the increased blood sugar monitoring you should do when you are adjusting your carb/insulin doses.

Increasing carbohydrate in your meals: how to adjust the insulin

If you are being taught insulin coverage for carbohydrate in the NHS or DAFNE courses, you will be taught that you simply use the same method as before.

30/units of insulin needed to cover this amount of carb to blood sugar target at any given meal = one unit of insulin will cover Xg of carb at this particular meal.

You would think that all you have to do is to divide the given number of carbs in the expected meal by this number to get your ideal insulin dose.

The problem is that the higher the carbohydrate content of the meal, the greater the insulin resistance that you will have so that you will actually need MORE insulin than calculated to achieve the same target blood sugar.

Instead of the linear relationship that you usually have with number of carbs eaten and number of units that need to be injected that exist in THOSE DIABETICS WHO ARE NOT INSULIN RESISTANT up to 30g of carbohydrate per meal, you will need progressively higher amounts of insulin injected after you eat more than 30g of carb for each meal.

As discussed earlier, the more insulin resistant you are, the more likely you are to need this extra whack of insulin, at even lower carb amounts than 30g.

This is because after 30g, or even before this, the graph is not linear, it is exponential.

How do you factor in the need for increasing insulin doses?

If you are really and truly perfectly happy to stick with 30g or less to each of your three meals a day, you do not need to learn and experiment with the following plan.

If, however, you WOULD like to eat higher carb meals either time to time or regularly, it is important that you figure out what you need to do so that your next pre-meal blood sugar is on target rather than wildly off.

Calculate insulin needed for 30g of carb and insulin sensitivity at each meal as previously.

Now calculate what you need to cover 40g of carb meals. Add to this 0.5 units of insulin. If you don't have half unit increment pens add 1 unit.

Eat this amount of carbohydrate, i.e. 40g at the meals you have chosen. Record the results for several meals.

Analyse your results. Did you hit the target bang on? Were your next meal blood sugars consistently low, possibly because you need less insulin than you calculated? Were you too high, perhaps because you require more insulin than you calculated?

Figure out how much extra insulin you need on top of your insulin sensitivity for 40g of carb meals. This could be different for breakfast, lunch and dinner.

You need to continue your experiments to find out exactly what insulin dose works for 40g meals, then 50g meals and so forth. I found that this worked fine with my son up till 90g per meal when the next meal blood sugars became unpredictable. This was before he hit his adolescent growth spurt and he was still quite insulin sensitive. Remember I told you about taking the nutritional scales into restaurants? You can see why. To make these experiments worthwhile you need to be sure of your carb quantities in the first place.

As soon as your experiments show that you cannot be predictable in your blood sugars even using this method, you have to accept that you CANNOT safely exceed that particular quantity of carb minus 10g for any given meal.

The meal that gives you the most forgiveness regarding this experiment is the weekend lunch. You will not be able to eat more carbs at any time of day and get away with it and have the time to sort yourself out before your evening meal and particularly bedtime. What you learn at these experiments can then be transferred to the rest of the week if you like.

If you love eating a particularly high carb dessert and you want to nail down the insulin dose, or be able to eat fettuccini Alfredo once a month, it is better to have that meal at lunch time.

You can continue meal experiments with all sorts of meals that have a mixture of protein, fat and carbohydrate. The technique is called meal profiling and you take your blood sugar one hour after completing each meal for five or more hours afterwards. You then see if you need more insulin to cover the first three hours, in which case you adjust the rapid acting insulin for the meal, or the later hours, in which case you need more regular insulin. If you ate four different breakfasts, seven different lunches and fourteen different evening meals, and it took four experiments to nail each one, you would have perfect blood sugars with meals in three months. At least, that is the theory. If you want to do this, again the best time to experiment is the lunch time meal at the weekend or when you have the day off.

Automated Bolus Calculators

There are now thousands of phone apps that can be used to help you calculate what dose of insulin you will need for a given amount of carbohydrate in a meal[81]. Some of the ones that are integrated into blood sugar meters are the Accu-chek Aviva Expert System and Freestyle InsuLinx.

They are a great help to diabetics for blood sugar/insulin management and work well for those who have figured out their individual meal/insulin sensitivities. The machines work on a linear calculation system. To be effective you need to be entirely CONSISTENT in the amount of carbs you are eating at each particular meal, whether that is low or moderate in carbs. They do not work that well for the sporadic high carb meal in a sea of low carb virtue.

CHAPTER SUMMARY

Again, there is a lot of information in this chapter and we appreciate that it will take time to understand and absorb. The basics are – read through all the group definitions and decide which one fits you best. You should then follow the guidelines for those groups when it comes to managing your medications and pairing this up with what you eat.

CHAPTER 7

CASE STUDIES

We have gone into some depth about working out what kind of blood sugar control you want to achieve and how you do it, but how does this work in real life? What about food preferences, driving, coping with being away from home, working out what to eat, working out how to adjust food and insulin by yourself?

Chances are it all feels rather overwhelming at the moment (we're sorry!) so to make life a little easier, here is a selection of different people with different needs and different blood sugar targets. Take a look at how the prescribed plan works for them.

Extremely tight blood sugar control: HbA1c 4.5-5.5% and daily carb intake 30-50g

Example 1. Dorothy is a 30-year-old type 1 diabetic woman who was diagnosed diabetic as a child. She has proliferative retinopathy. Dorothy takes insulin to control her diabetes – fast-acting insulin, regular insulin and basal insulin (long-acting insulin).

She has progressively tightened up on her blood sugars over the last year and is now ready for the big push to get normal blood sugar control because she would like to get pregnant. She eats 10g of carbohydrate for each meal and a bedtime snack of 10g – so a daily intake of 40g.

A typical day's meal is

1. Breakfast is 3 boiled eggs and a low carb muffin. 10g carbs

2. Lunch is a chicken salad, followed by berries and double cream. 10g carbs

3. Dinner is lamb stew with carrots, celery and onions. 10g carbs

4. Bedtime she eats cheddar cheese, a mini oatcake 2g butter and half an apple. 8g

Dorothy asks: "I've never been on as little insulin as this since I was diagnosed. How do I calculate the exact doses I need and make sure I don't get low blood sugars overnight?"

To calculate her insulin doses, Dorothy needs to know her carbohydrate sensitivity for each meal.

She has worked out that one unit of rapid acting insulin will cover 7g of carb at breakfast, 10g of carb at lunch, 9g of carb in the evening, and for safety regarding night blood sugars, she should give 2/3 of the dose of insulin for her night time snack as she does for her evening meal, that is one unit to cover 12g of carbohydrate rather than the 9g for her evening meal.

The straightforward calculation is to add on one-third of the carbohydrate to what you would usually cover with the evening dose of insulin.

Now she needs to work out how much protein she is eating at each meal. Pen users would cover this with their regular insulin. For ease of calculation, stick to the same protein sensitivity coverage at each meal. We use ounces to estimate protein and grams to determine carbohydrate.

1. 3 boiled eggs = 3oz protein = 2 units

2. One chicken breast = 6oz 6/3 x 2 = 4 units regular insulin. Give 4 units.

3. Lamb stew (meat only) 5oz 5/3 x 2 = 3.3 units. Give 3 units.

4. There is not enough protein in the cheese to merit coverage with insulin.

She has already adjusted her dietary carbohydrate so that she IS eating a very low-carb diet of approximately 10g for each meal.

Breakfast one unit of insulin covers 7 grams carb. To cover 10g carb, she needs 10/7 = 1.4 units of rapid acting insulin. Give 1.5 units.

Lunch one unit of insulin covers 10g carb. To cover 10g, she needs one unit of rapid acting insulin.

Dinner one unit of insulin covers 9g carb. 10/9 = 1.1 units of insulin. Give one unit.

Bedtime snack one unit of insulin covers 12g carb. 10/12 = 0.83 units insulin. Give 0.5 units. (Always err on the side of lower insulin doses over the period of time that covers night time).

You can see that her meal insulin doses will be:

1. Breakfast 2 units regular insulin and 1.5 units rapid acting insulin.

2. Lunch 4 units regular insulin and one unit rapid acting insulin.

3. Evening meal 3 units regular insulin and one unit rapid-acting insulin.

4. Before bed 0.5 units of rapid acting insulin.

5. She would also take her basal insulin on rising and before bed.

Example 2: Janice is a 48-year-old woman who has newly been diagnosed with type 2 diabetes. Her mother is also diabetic, type 2, on insulin, who has had an amputation thanks to the effects of diabetes. Janice is terrified of the same thing happening to her. She is keen to get her blood sugars as normal as possible.

She eats for breakfast:

1. Bacon, fried eggs, mushrooms 5g and tomato 5g (10g total)

2. Lunch is roast beef, horseradish sauce, green salad, and a plum, 15g total

3. Dinner is sole fried in butter and olive oil, cauliflower mash 5g and three squares of dark chocolate (15g total).

She asks: "I'm new to carb counting. What is the easiest way to learn it?"

The easiest way to learn carb counting is probably to stick to foods that you know are really low in carbohydrate. These are non-starchy vegetables, and you will base your meals around protein (fish, meat, eggs, poultry and tofu) padded out with these vegetables.

A simple way to pick out the vegetables that you are going to eat or not is to look at the Collins Gem Carb counting book. Run your eye down the "net carb"[82] column and see what comes in at under 5g for a small portion: asparagus, aubergine, avocado, bamboo shoots, French beans, runner beans, green beans, bean sprouts, beetroot, broccoli, cabbage, spring greens, carrots, cauliflower, celeriac, celery, chicory, courgettes, fennel, garlic, ginger, gherkins, kale, kohlrabi, leeks, lettuce, mange tout, marrow, mushrooms, okra, olives, onions, peppers, pumpkin, radishes, spinach, spring onions, squash, swede, tomatoes, turnip, and water chestnuts.

Example 3. Mary is a type 2 diabetic who was on maximal oral therapy with an HbA1c of 10.5%. She was started on insulin, a basal-bolus regime and, at the same time, started a strict low-carb diet of 50g a day.

This was mainly to reduce the amount of insulin she had to inject and also to reverse any complications. Her blood sugars had been running high for about four years, but she had been afraid to start insulin. Her HbA1c is now 4.8% with no hypos because her pancreas is doing the fine-tuning.

1. Breakfast is: a vegetable omelette (mushroom, pepper, spring onion) and an orange 20g carbs

2. Lunch is meatballs, tomato sauce, and creamed spinach, 10g carbs

3. Dinner is roast chicken, cabbage 5g and butter with a slice of low carb Victoria sponge, 15g carbs.

Mary asks: "How do I adjust my insulins based on my blood sugar test results throughout the day?"

Mary has three different insulins – basal (long-acting), regular and rapid.

The basal insulin (Levemir®) lasts about 14 hours and is given twice a day. One injection is given just before her breakfast in the morning, and the other is given before bedtime at night. She gives the same dose of it each time.

She bases the dose on her 2-4am blood sugar test which she does once a week. She could test it more often as she gets up to pass urine at night more often than this. She aims to get the blood sugar level at these times to be between 4.0 and 6.0.

If she gets lower than 4.0 through the night, she CUTS the dose of Levemir® both morning and night by one unit each and repeats the 2-4am test two nights later.

If her 2-4am blood sugar level gets higher than 6.0, she repeats the test two nights later and only increases the dose of Levemir® by one unit both morning and night if this too is elevated.

Her regular insulin is only used to cover protein. She keeps to the formula two units of regular insulin for every 3oz /90g portion of meat. This never changes.

She uses rapid insulin to cover dietary carbohydrate and for correction doses if she has an unexpectedly high blood sugar (over 10mmol).

The formula for correction doses of insulin in a NON-insulin resistant adult is one unit of NovoRapid (rapid-acting insulin), which will drop your blood sugar by 2.5 mmol/l in 1-2 hours.

For those people with significant insulin resistance, they will need more insulin than this, often double the amount of insulin for the same drop in blood-sugar levels.

Small people (less body weight) and children will need a lot less insulin for the same drop in blood sugar levels. You need to keep records to see just how your blood sugar responds.

If you have a cold, the flu or other illness, you will often become temporarily insulin resistant and may need very high doses of insulin to take down a high blood sugar. If this happens, you should check your blood sugars every 2½ hours and tailor your correction insulin doses to your response.

For carbohydrate in her meals, Mary uses the rapid-acting insulin. To know exactly how much insulin she needs to inject, she also needs to know her insulin sensitivity. She can work this out by deciding to eat the same number of carbohydrates for each meal every day for a week and adjusting the amount of insulin she gives the next day for the same meal according to how accurately she hit her blood sugar targets before the following meal. Ideally, she would have very similar types of meals.

The three-day food diary/blood sugar sheets that are available online in the appendix are very helpful here.

Breakfast every day: one vegetable, 2-egg omelette and one small/medium piece of fruit. 15 g carbs.

DAY	BLOOD SUGAR LEVEL BEFORE BREAKFAST	MORNING INSULIN DOSE TO COVER BREAKFAST	BLOOD SUGAR LEVEL BEFORE LUNCH
MONDAY	7.2	4	3.4 (too low)
TUESDAY	6.5	3.5	4.8 (on target)
WEDNESDAY	9.0	4 (larger dose than yesterday to cover higher than normal morning blood sugar levels)	5.2 (on target)
THURSDAY	7.8	3.5	5.2 (on target)

Of the useful tests, 4 units are bringing the blood sugar level a bit too low before the next meal, but 3.5 units are on target twice. On Wednesday, the first am blood sugar is a bit higher than the others, so Mary won't know if her meal dose is going to be accurate as she has to guess for a correction dose as well.

Her insulin sensitivity for breakfast is 15g/3.5 units, i.e. one unit will cover 4.2 g of carb at breakfast. It is reasonable to average this to one unit of carb at breakfast will cover 4g of carb.

Once Mary knows this, she can take a better guess at what her likely insulin sensitivity at lunch time will be. Her insulin sensitivity will generally be better than at breakfast because the dawn phenomenon is no longer active. She could then experiment with giving one unit of insulin for 5g of carb or 6g of carb or even 7g of carb at lunch. By experimentation, she can find out exactly what amounts of insulin she needs for a particular carb count at each meal.

Tight blood sugar control: HbA1c 5.5-6.5 carb intake 50-90g

Example 1. David is a type 1 diabetic aged 22. He is a post-graduate student who cooks for himself and eats out a lot. He has had diabetes for 10 years, has no complications and wants to keep it that way.

1. He eats for breakfast: peanut choc chip cookies (low carb), 2 slices of cold ham. One apple.

2. Lunch is burger, cheese, salad, mayo, ketchup (no bun)

3. Dinner is chicken caesar salad, ice cream.

David asks: "When is the optimal time to inject my insulin to cover my meals, and to cope with insulin injections when eating out?"

For meal coverage, the optimal time to inject rapid and regular insulins is 15-30 minutes before a meal if your pre-meal blood sugar target is 4-7 mmol/l[83] .

Realistically, David will only manage the 30-minute before-hand injection if he is at home and knows what he is having and how much carbohydrate he intends to eat.

In restaurants, he can inject insulin once his order has been taken. He may not know exactly how much he is going to eat, but he can inject up to 7 units of regular insulin for the protein component and up to 7 units for the carbohydrate component and make up any additional insulin as needed once he has eyeballed the meal or actually eaten it.

Before he injects, he has to ask for bread to be brought to the table in case the meal is delayed and he gets a hypo because of the insulin he has taken.

Most food in restaurants takes 20-40 minutes to arrive for main courses ordered on their own. If you order a starter, you usually get these within 10 minutes. Starters are often low carb and usually don't come with the rice, potatoes, pasta and pastry that accompany mains[84]. Often ordering two starters instead of a main meal can work well.

Should David have a blood sugar under 4, he is best not to inject any insulin until he has eaten some of his meal. He would then inject the required amount of insulin or somewhat less than the calculation would suggest.

If his blood sugar is over 7, he will factor in a correction dose and give this along with the meal insulin. The standard correction dose is one unit of rapid acting insulin for every 2.5mmol blood sugar drop required. If blood sugar is high, it is also advisable to eat a starter which is particularly low in carbs. This gives the insulin time to get absorbed and start to bring the blood sugars down. These items include olives, pate, prawns and cold meats.

Example 2. Robin is a newly diagnosed type 1 diabetic aged 28. He runs a shop and has to drive a lot. He gets great deals on out of date luxury food.

1. He eats for breakfast: low-carb cheesecake, cream, strawberries.

2. Lunch: smoked salmon, cream cheese, onion, a pear.

3. Dinner: roast lamb, broccoli in cheese sauce. Low carb chocolate mousse.

Robin asks: "I want to exercise, but I don't know the best way to manage my insulin injections for this. It is very important that I don't get hypos as I need to drive for my job."

Insulin users are best to exercise at the same time every day so they can get into a smooth routine with their basal insulin, diet and meal insulin. For someone with a regular shift pattern, they can work out what time of day is best for them to exercise and work around that. The time chosen may vary according to whether the shift changes or not.

For strenuous or prolonged exercise Robin has to decide whether he will cut his basal insulin, cut his meal insulin or eat extra carbohydrate. Although all exercisers need to have rapid acting carb available when and after they exercise, it will be counterproductive to eat extra carb if you are trying to lose weight. Therefore, cutting insulin in a planned way will be needed.

If blood sugars are particularly high, over 11mmol, it is best not to exercise before this is brought down by a correction dose of insulin. Some people's blood sugars can go up with exercise. Gentle walking, in general, lowers blood sugars, and this can be especially useful after meals. Sprinting and other forms of high-intensity exercise, however, raise your blood sugar. Any competitive sport where cortisol is released is also likely to raise blood sugars. Weight training beyond 45-60 minutes a day can also result in a rise in cortisol and thus raise blood sugars.

As always with diabetes, you have to see what your blood sugar patterns are and guess what the best thing to do would be. Then do it next time and look at the results you get and analyse again. Women have the added difficulty of variation in insulin resistance at different phases of their menstrual cycles to contend with.

As Robin drives, he needs to take extra precautions to avoid hypoglycaemia with exercise. He needs to keep glucose in the car and check his blood sugar before setting off and after every hour of driving.

Example 3. Colin is a 65-year-old retired man who has diabetic retinopathy, for which he has been getting laser treatment. He has had type two diabetes for 15 years. His HbA1c has been around 7-8.5% for most of this time.

He has heard about low carbing as an effective treatment for diabetes. He cut down his carbs gradually till he was at 90g of carb a day. His oral hypoglycaemics and other drugs were reduced but not stopped. His retinopathy halted in its tracks, and he knows he has to keep to this level of restriction long-term.

1. He eats scrambled eggs, smoked salmon, tomato. One slice of toast.

2. Lunch: chilli con carne with kidney beans, fruit salad, cream.

3. Dinner: lentil soup, sea bass, green beans, cheese, apple.

He asks: "I have friends over for meals quite a lot. How do I work out the meals so that I keep to my diet, but they don't feel deprived?"

The main thing to do to please your non-low carbing friends and yourself is to have meals where carbohydrates are not the main component and meals where carbohydrates can be easily separated out from the meal.

Coeliacs have to be particularly careful in this regard with wheat avoidance.

Starters:

1. Avoid soups with rice, pasta and potatoes in them. Provide bread and butter with soups instead. Make homemade soups and serve with cream.

2. Many fish, seafood, thinly sliced meat and olives and other vegetables can be served with bread on the side.

Mains:

Avoid combination meals such as lasagne unless the pasta is replaced with vegetables such as courgettes or leeks. You can serve many different roast types of meat, fish, seafood, and stews and serve a risotto, pasta, or potato dish on the side. You can have plenty of vegetables also on the side so that people can help themselves and get the quantities of individual items that suit them.

You can make meals with cauliflower mash instead of potatoes. Many guests will be perfectly happy with this. Cheese sauces can be done with double cream and grated cheddar cheese instead of flour. Grated cauliflower that has been gently steamed can substitute to some extent for rice.

Desserts:

Cheese and fruit can be served with biscuits on the side.

You can make low carb or high-carb desserts and serve them in individual containers. Examples could be chocolate mousses, custards and panna cotta. Many low-carb cakes and cheesecakes are superb.

Even low carb shortcrust pastry can be made, and this can be the base for both cheesecakes and open or closed fruit pies.

Low carb pancakes and low carb ice cream are also possible. It is easy to provide a commercially produced dessert but stick to the cheese and fruit yourself.

Irish coffees need to be made with real sugar to get the cream to float properly. You won't be able to have one yourself if you are seriously low carbing.

Pure spirits and some cocktails are better regarding carbs. One low carb cookbook has a low-carb cocktail section, which the writer prefers to desserts. (*A Passion for Protein* by Henry Harris.)

Good enough control: HbA1c 6-7% carb intake 90-120g

Example 1. Marjorie is a 58-year-old newly-diagnosed type 2 diabetic. She is very overweight, and her baseline HbA1c is 10.5%. After two months on this diet, her HbA1c is 6.8%, and she has lost 2 stones. She initially started on a lower carb target than this but missed carbohydrates a lot.

1. She eats for breakfast, smoked mackerel, fruit salad, Greek yoghurt.

2. Lunch: 2 oatcakes, butter, chicken liver pate and two satsumas.

3. Dinner: Steak, mushroom and cream sauce, a small portion of boiled rice.

She asks: "I bought a nutritional scale to help me count carbohydrates. How do I use it?"

Nutritional scales cost from £10-40. They work by weighing the food in the portion you intend to eat and putting in a code either from a book provided or, in more expensive scales, by selecting the food item from an inbuilt computer.

Marjorie would start by selecting the items from her diet that have a substantial amount of carbohydrate in them and then testing these on the scale. Once she has done this for a while, she will quickly get an idea of how many grams of carbs different food contains from just looking at the portion size. To start with, measuring gets your carb counting skills off to a good start.

At breakfast, the carb-containing items are the fruit salad and yoghurt. Mackerel is a protein.

Marjorie has made her own fruit salad, so there is no entry for it in the book supplied. It contains, apple, orange, melon and strawberries. Melon and strawberries tend to be lower in sugars than apples and oranges, so Marjorie picks the fruit that seems middle of the road which is probably apple and puts this into the computer.

Apples peeled and sliced have the code 205. She switches on the scale, selects grams, and puts in the code. The carb count comes up as 20.

She now wants to count the carb in the yoghurt. There is no code for Greek style yoghurt in the book. She looks up her Collins Gem Carb counter and sees that a 125g pot of this has 6g of carb. She intends to eat half of the 250g pot, so now has a total breakfast carb count of 26g.

At lunch, the carbohydrate containing items are the oatcakes and the satsumas. The pate is a mixture of fat and protein. The oatcakes are listed as 5g each on the packet so these account for 10g. The satsumas code is 289. The carb count comes up as 15g. Her total lunch carb is therefore 25g.

At dinner, Marjorie could weigh the mushrooms before she makes the sauce. The code for these is 875. The carb count is 4. She now measures the rice. The code for long grain uncooked rice is 483. The carb count is 60.

As she goes along Marjorie will notice that it is a lot more important to weigh high carb items like rice, potatoes and pasta compared to low starch vegetables such as mushrooms, asparagus and broccoli.

Her daily total is 115g carbs, which is just within the target she has set for herself.

Example 2. Richard is seven years old, a type one diabetic and he takes a packed lunch to school. His mother is happy that his blood sugars are, while not perfect, a lot better than average. He can eat the same sort of food at school as his mates.

1. He eats for breakfast: 2 sausages, baked beans, 1 fried egg.
2. For lunch: roast chicken sandwiches, a packet of crisps, and an apple.
3. For dinner: mince, sweet corn, peas.

Richard's mum, Lisa, asks: "What should I do to smooth the way for Richard's diabetes management at school?"

Lisa has two main routes to help Richard at school with his diabetes management. She can go to the school directly, or she can involve the diabetic liaison nurse from the hospital to visit. I would suggest doing both.

Lisa needs to speak to the head teacher of the school and seek permission to talk to the class teacher, Physical Education teacher and school nurse.

Regarding day-to-day management, Richard needs to be able to test his blood sugar at his desk whenever he thinks he may be having a hypo. He needs to be able to snack in class if his blood sugar is low. He needs to carry sweets for this. Basset's Jelly Babies, e.g. have 4.2g of carb each and 3 or 4 of these will usually raise the blood sugar well.

Richard needs to be able to inject insulin in the canteen. It is not appropriate to ask him to test and inject only in the toilets. (This has happened!)

He is more at risk of hypos during or after PE, so the teachers need to be able to recognise signs of low blood sugar. They then need to be able to ask him to test and treat if appropriate. Often diabetics have their own particular symptoms of low blood sugar. Lisa needs to tell them what these are so they can intervene early if they spot Richard experiencing these signs.

The Insulin Dependent Diabetes Trust has advice to parents and teacher about looking after school age children with diabetes. Diabetes UK runs camps for children under the age of 12 and his or her parent.

Signs of low blood sugar can include:

1. Pallor

2. Sweating

3. Bad temper

4. Shaking

5. Feeling cold

6. Poor vision

7. Incoordination

8. Loss of concentration

Example 3: Deanne is an 18-year-old girl who has type two diabetes. She has a family history of this, and she is also very overweight. She finds it embarrassing to go to a gym but has started walking with a group at college. She loves chocolate and pizza.

1. She eats for breakfast: low carb pancakes and butter. Blueberries.

2. Lunch: 2 slices of pizza, side salad.

3. Dinner: Gammon steak, pineapple, courgettes, butter. Dark chocolate with nuts.

She asks: "How do I manage my food cravings?"

Food cravings can be due to various things. One important one is downright hunger. You can get this under control by eating enough protein at meals. If necessary, eat more protein or protein/fat snacks between meals, especially nuts as they can tide you over until the next meal. This may have some importance if there is a large gap between lunch and the evening meal.

Low blood sugars brought on by excessive insulin secretion from dealing with the last meal can make you feel hungry. Cutting down the amount of sugar and starch at all meals can help.

Chromium supplementation may help type 2s[85]. This mineral has been shown to help in some studies, but not in others.

High sugar, fat and salt foods can be addictive because they are hyper-palatable foods. So can caffeine. Do you crave a particular thing – we're going to guess you are more likely to report cravings for crisps, chocolate or ice-cream, rather than a desire to eat unlimited amounts of steak?

Breaking the crisp/chocolate habit can be hard. Probably the best thing to do is to replace it with some activity or foodstuffs that are less damaging to your weight and blood sugars. Exercise, eating raw vegetables, or knitting for instance. Easier said than done, we know, but another key tactic for dealing with craving is not to keep your food of over-eating choice in the house.

Is eating in front of the TV the problem?

When you eat without giving due attention to where and how you eat it, you will probably end up overeating. You will tend to eat more quickly and forget just how much you put away. It is best to eat meals at a table, sitting down and eat slowly. It takes your brain 20 minutes to catch up with your stomach and for the hunger hormones to subside. Sometimes just some "eating hygiene" is all you need.

Do you eat from plain boredom?

"Oh, what will I do with myself? Tea and biscuits? That sounds great..." Five biscuits later and you are still bored, unfortunately, but you are now also coping with high blood sugars from those biscuits. Eating out of boredom is one of most common forms of emotional eating – and eating for reasons such as this never solves the original problem.

If you have time on your hands, work out what you really enjoy doing, or what gives you a sense of satisfaction. Giving yourself a manicure/pedicure, tidying cupboards, washing windows, writing or phoning friends, playing with your cat, taking your dog or the neighbour's dog out for a walk, or craft work would all be better for your blood sugar than eating.

Do you need to eat when you drink?

The song says, "Love and marriage go together like a horse and carriage." Is this how you view coffee and biscuits? Tea and cake? Coke and popcorn? Milk shake and a burger? If you can learn to drink and not eat at the same time, it can free you from a multitude of snack calories.

Do you eat just because other people are doing it?

It can be hard to keep your hand out of the chocolate box when it has been brought in "as a treat" to your workplace, and everyone else is getting stuck in. Sometimes not eating is seen as downright unsociable. Can you join in by just having a low cal drink instead? Can you just deploy, the "it doesn't agree with me" excuse? Will anyone really be bothered if you don't eat it? Does it matter to you if they are?

For more information on eating habits and self-esteem, see Appendix H.

Looser control: HbA1c 7-8% carb intake 120-150g

Example 1. Peter is a 70-year-old man who has been a very overweight type 2 diabetic for many years. He is on Victoza injections, and this helps control his appetite. He has no complications apart from some tendon stiffening in his shoulders and legs.

1. He eats for breakfast: cornflakes, milk, scrambled eggs with cheese.

2. Lunch: vegetable soup, roast pork sandwich, cherries.

3. Dinner: stir fried chicken, carrots, courgettes and onion. Ice cream.

He asks: "How do I use 'carb factors' to count the carbohydrates I am eating?"

The carbohydrate factor of food is the percent of the food's total weight that is carbohydrate. Multiply the weight of a portion of food in grams by its carbohydrate factor to find the number of grams of carbohydrate in it. You need a scale that accurately counts in grams. Simply weigh the food. For every 100g of that particular food, you get the values seen, e.g. 100g worth of bagel = 56g carbs.

For a list of carbohydrate factors, see Appendix H. According to the list, Peter's breakfast carb items are cornflakes with milk. He puts out a small portion of cornflakes of 60g and finds that the carb for this is 84 x 60%= 50g. Milk is 10g for a glass. His total breakfast carb is 60g.

His lunch carbs are the vegetable soup, bread in his sandwich and the cherries. Vegetable soup is not on this list (although he will be able to find it on the internet at the USDA site). Collins Gems gives a carb count of 15g for 200mls of Baxters Chunky vegetable soup.

Bread has a carb factor of 0.53. It is worth knowing that the carb factor of most soft baked goods is around 0.5. This means that if you can weigh an item, you get 50g of carb for every 100g of the product. This is a rule of thumb that can help if you don't have access to carb factors. He weighs the bread. It is 90g. 90% of 53g is 47g.

He looks up the USDA site and searches for cherries. He finds that 100g of cherries (before being stoned) come in at 12g of carb. He weighs out 100g. His total lunch carb is therefore 74g.

For dinner, his carb items are carrots, courgettes, onion and then ice cream. He has 100g of carrots which have a carb factor of 0.07. These, therefore, come in at 7g of carb. Courgettes seem to be unlisted, but under their American name of Zucchini they come up as summer squash. Their carb factor is 0.03 making 100g have a carb count of only 3. Onions in the USDA tables come in at 9g of carb for every 100g. He is having 50g, so the carb count is 4.5g.

Ice cream is not listed in the table but is found on the USDA website. It is 29g carb for every 100g. Helpfully a half cup serving of 76g is suggested, and this has a carb count of 22g. This would be the amount of only one scoop, which is a useful measurement to remember for days out.

Peter's total meal count for dinner is therefore 36.5g.

Example 2. Lynn is a 35-year-old woman who has had type 1 diabetes from childhood. She has had "average" control with HbA1cs in the 8-10% range for many years. She has proliferative retinopathy and has had laser treatment on her eyes several times.

Unfortunately, she developed multiple sclerosis aged 28, and this has pursued a very aggressive course. She is on treatment with toxic drugs that affect her autoimmune system, but despite this, she is having great difficulty walking and is in a lot of pain. She cannot exercise.

1. She eats for breakfast: sugar-free muesli with milk, prunes.

2. For lunch: prawn cocktail, vegetable soup and an apple.

3. For dinner: mushroom risotto, cheese.

Lynn asks: "I sometimes wonder if my life is worth living. What is the point of trying for reasonable blood sugars when I feel so miserable?"

Many people with diabetes get fed up with the demands of looking after their condition. Let's face it, life is pretty tough, and the added burden of looking after yourself when you have an additional serious medical problem can sometimes feel intolerable. When you have diabetes you often have to eat differently to other people, you need to check blood sugars frequently, act on the results and exercise consistently.

Also, you can never "just have a cold", because if you are not careful, it can escalate into ketoacidosis if you are type 1, or escalate into a serious chest infection if your immune system is not functioning as well as it should with type 2.

A major issue is that if you just give up with your diabetes management things can and will get a hell of a lot worse. High blood sugars affect your energy, concentration and memory, low blood sugars affect your confidence and swinging blood sugars affect your moods. Immediate problems such as infection can get a lot worse with high blood sugars and even minor skin problems associated with diabetes can change your appearance and impair your sleep.

Multiple sclerosis has some similarities with diabetic neuropathy because the nervous system becomes damaged in both conditions. Pain, weakness, and numbness can affect mobility for both. In general, the drug treatments for diabetes are much less toxic than for MS. It can seem just so unfair to have two serious problems and depression to contend with.

Lynn needs to get as much practical help as she can:

Is she getting all the benefits she is entitled to? A referral to a social worker could help here.

Would aids in the house help? A referral to an occupational therapist may help.

Should she get a wheelchair that would help her get out and about? Many people with diabetes and neurological conditions see being in a wheelchair as a last resort, but using this aid can improve your social life and reduce the tiredness associated with the degree of physical exertion that is required to walk.

Physiotherapists can maximise functional ability and keep limbs as strong and supple as possible.

Everyone has emotional needs as well as physical needs. This is a list that psychotherapists use to assess mental well-being. Are your emotional needs not being met? Everyone needs these fulfilled most of the time to stay calm and productive.

1. A sense of control over day to day events

2. Able to relax when needing to

3. Able to give attention to others

4. Feeling that life is meaningful

5. Interest and pleasure in doing things

6. Able to stay calm in challenging situations

7. Having enough time and space for yourself

8. Feeling safe and secure

9. Getting enough sleep

10. Feeling closeness or connected to someone

11. Feeling positive and hopeful

12. Able to deal with problems effectively

13. Able to achieve something

14. Feeling valued and respected

15. Getting positive attention from others.

Referral for counselling or psychological therapy may be accessed from a visit to your GP.

Do you think you have depression? This test helps you figure out if you do and what type it may be: www.depressedtest.com/

If you think you have a problem, please see your GP or psychologist at your diabetic clinic.

If the GP or hospital specialist is not able to improve the different types of pain that people with diabetes and multiple sclerosis tend to have, they can refer to a pain clinic. These are usually run by anaesthetists, and they can suggest alternative medication and nerve blocks.

Exercises can improve mood and reduce the perception of pain. Lynn may need to get special chair exercise videos.

Example 3. Debbie is a 14-year-old type 1 diabetic. She is not far from the peak of her insulin resistance, and it is to be expected that her blood sugars will be erratic for at least another three or four years. She doesn't mind eating lower carb at home, but does want to eat the same as her friends at school and when she goes out with them. Even though Debbie eats at the lower end of the carb scale for this group, her HbA1c is at the top end.

1. She eats for breakfast: smoked salmon, scrambled eggs, tomato.

2. Lunch: pasta, tomato sauce. Crisps. Chocolate biscuit.

3. Dinner: low carb moussaka, salad.

Debbie asks: "How am I ever going to manage to go away to university with diabetes? I'm going to be stuck at home with my mum and dad forever."

Debbie is almost at the peak age for insulin resistance in teenage girls, and her blood sugar control will usually be near its worst at this point. It is easy to lose heart. By the time she is 17 or 18, however, she will be able to use less insulin to gain blood sugar control than she does now, and the dawn phenomenon will not be as pronounced. Meanwhile, she just has to keep going. It really will be much better as she approaches time to go to university.

She has the added problem of the high blood sugars that are typical on the run up to menstruation. It would be worth considering a method of contraception that gives hormonal stability throughout the cycle such as Cerazette or Loestrin 20 every day. This is discussed further in the FAQ section.

Planning about how to arrange the transition between home and life away at university is well worth while. Debbie and her parents can then plan a gradual removal of responsibility for diabetic management and other tasks over a period of 3 or 4 years. It should be remembered that non-diabetic students also struggle with life away from home particularly if mum has done all their washing, shopping, financial management, cleaning and cooking prior to the big day.

Regarding the non-diabetic related things, it would be worth getting Debbie her own bank account and putting money in it monthly so she can budget for her own clothes, footwear, hairdressing and other expenses. She should get an alarm clock and get herself up in the mornings.

Debbie should learn how to clean a house, do the laundry, budget for food shopping and learn to make simple meals for the whole family one or more times a week. She would benefit from learning to bake the low carb way so her diet can be both low in carb and enjoyable.

She can get a provisional driving licence from the age of 17 and might wish to take driving lessons and sit the tests during the long summer holidays before university starts or at some point in her course. Alternatively, she may want to undertake work experience. This is an essential part of the admissions process for some courses.

As far as diabetes management goes, she needs to learn all about how to get as normal blood sugars as she can from this book and other resources we mention. She should consider obtaining and using a bolus calculator system such as the Aviva Expert System or an insulin pump if she prefers.

She has to become responsible for checking her own blood sugars at least before every meal, before bed, and more often if undertaking exercise, during illness or if she doesn't feel right or if her friends and family ask her to test to see if she is having low blood sugars. It is well worth learning how to cover higher carb items such as pizza, spaghetti and chips. Although we do not recommend these foods for regular consumption, they can be hard to avoid when you are a student.

She needs to learn to carb count accurately at home and learn to "eyeball" portions when outside the house.

She will soon be seeing doctors and other health professionals on her own, but she needs to discuss any change in management with her parents. She needs to attend for eye and foot checks and get her flu immunisation done from every October onwards.

She should mention in her university application that she has type 1 diabetes. This counts as a disability. She is more likely to be placed in a hall of residence for the first and even second year if she has this on her form. She also needs to have access to a fridge where she can store her insulin and food.

One family I know had their daughter lodge with a family friend for her sixth year. Although the houses were only a short car ride away, this gave their daughter the experience of living away from home and looking after her own diabetes.

Debbie should have a copy of her relevant medical notes. In the UK, her GP can give her a copy of her intermediate summary and a copy of the most important diabetic clinic letters and blood results. She can take a copy of this to her new GP and also have it with her if an on-call GP needs to see her at any time or she needs to go to A and E.

She should be allocated a room near a kitchen, but should specifically mention that she needs this.

She should visit the pharmacy that she intends to use at the university and introduce herself. Pharmacists will usually dispense insulin in an emergency without a prescription if there has been some sort of hold up. She should keep a copy of her repeat prescriptions in a special green cross marked tub in the fridge of her residence and at home. This is where paramedics have been trained to look. You put a green cross on the door of the flat, so they know it is there. These are obtainable from a pharmacy.

Debbie will need to obtain her own repeat prescriptions and know how to dispose of her yellow sharps bin where she will dispose of her needles and lancets. She takes it to the pharmacist.

If you have a type 1 diabetic son or daughter who is about to go to university or college or leave home, then it is worth your while to take your son or daughter's new flat mates out to dinner and explain how to recognise and treat hypos, sick day rules, and diabetic ketoacidosis[86]. The management will range from asking Debbie to check her blood sugar to calling you, calling her GP/out of hours service and calling 999. Give a note of all your contact numbers so it can go on a notice board in the flat so you can be contacted at any time.

Setting up Skype on your respective computers can be a cheap and effective way of keeping in regular contact.

The new GP can arrange hospital appointments and Debbie herself can phone up to speak to the diabetic liaison nurse.

CHAPTER SUMMARY

As you will have read, there are lots of different situations that apply to people with diabetes and a lot of different considerations to take into account. We have covered carbohydrate counting, insulin adjusting, dining out, cooking for friends, coping with food cravings, dealing with depression, exercising and driving, but this list is not exhaustive. What it should have shown you though, is how to live with diabetes in different situations, one of which will hopefully resemble your own.

As a reminder, the definitions are:

Extremely tight blood sugar control – 4.5-5.5% HbA1c (good for women who are planning a pregnancy, women who are pregnant and who are not achieving an HbA1c even on meals of 30g carbs, people who are still suffering from troublesome hypos, and young adults who have diabetes-related complications they wish to reverse)

Tight blood sugar control – 5.5 to 6.5% HbA1c (suitable for older children, newly diagnosed diabetics (type 1 and type 2s, pregnant women and those planning a pregnancy and experienced insulin pumpers)

"Good enough" blood sugar control – 6.5-7% HbA1c (good for people who drive a lot, late middle-aged type 2 diabetics with no complications, those new to insulin pumps and individuals with proliferative retinopathy or peripheral neuropathy)

Looser blood sugar control – 7-8% HbA1c (for babies and toddlers, adolescent girls and older diabetics).

CHAPTER 8

FREQUENTLY ASKED QUESTIONS

B y this stage of the book, your head may well be buzzing with all of the information we have presented to you.

Fear not! We have pulled together what we think are the frequently asked questions of the low-carb-eating-living-with-diabetes community so read on to find the answers to (hopefully) all of your questions...

Q. How do I lower my blood sugar if it is running too high?

A. Dr Katharine Morrison: If you use insulin you can use correction doses of rapid acting insulin to bring down a high blood sugar. For non-insulin resistant adults, the rule of thumb is that one unit of rapid acting insulin will lower your blood sugar by 2.5mmol/l (45mg). Thus, if your blood sugar is 10mmol/l (180mg) and you want to bring it down to 5mmol/l (90mg), you would inject two units of your rapid acting insulin.

If you are particularly small framed or a child you will need LESS insulin than this to bring your blood sugar down. If you are very insulin resistant, e.g. an adolescent or you have metabolic syndrome the amount of insulin needed will be MORE. When my son was at peak insulin resistance aged 16 he needed more like one unit of rapid acting insulin to bring his blood sugar levels down by one mmol/l.

Q. What is the best way to treat a hypo (low blood sugar levels)?

A. Dr Katharine Morrison: Use a pure glucose preparation to deal with a hypo. 15g worth of glucose tablets, Lucozade, or liquid glucose is the fastest way to get your blood sugar up. Because glucose tablets, Lucozade and liquid glucose bring your blood glucose level up quickly, you are less likely to over treat yourself with high amounts of carbohydrate, so you end up with a very high blood sugar. If you treat yourself with a chocolate bar, for example, then it might not act quickly enough, and you may end up eating too many carbohydrates.

Emma Baird: And read my note in Chapter 3 on horrible hypos and the dangers of over-treating! I like using jelly babies to treat my hypos as they are easy to find. You can buy them in practically every shop – from the newsagent to the garage, to the off-licence, supermarkets and even DIY stores. Four jelly babies usually do the trick.

Q. How do I get my GP and diabetologist to accept that I want to get normal blood sugars and eat a low carb diet?

A. Dr Katharine Morrison: I have found it very difficult to get fellow GPs and diabetologists round to thinking that normal blood sugars are a fundamental right for diabetics and that it is perfectly achievable on a low carb diet too!

However, a way to influence your doctor is to ask him or her to MONITOR your results. This has been found to be a very successful strategy by a bariatric physician and co-author of the Atkins Diabetes Revolution, Dr Mary Vernon from Kansas.[87] Dr Vernon has found that doctors are usually happy to do the same sort of tests as they usually do and pass on the results to the patient as long as the patient takes responsibility for their diet and blood sugar management.

By monitoring your results, what I mean is that you ask your doctor or diabetologist to keep note of key information such as your blood pressure, triglyceride levels, HbA1C, waist size, HDL and LDL levels. If you stick to your low carbohydrate diet, these figures should all improve – and voila, this ought to persuade your doctors that what you are doing is right.

THE ANTI LOW CARBERS

"So why are dieticians and doctors against the low-carbohydrate diet?"

Dieticians, in particular, have been trained to believe that eating a high-fat diet, particularly saturated fat, causes heart disease. It does not. (See the answer to the question about saturated fat for more on this subject).

Training for doctors in nutrition at medical school is minimal. They are taught very little about PREVENTION of disease and much more about DIAGNOSIS and TREATMENT. In my experience at medical school, I was also taught a lot more about unusual diseases than about common diseases, writes Dr Katharine Morrison.

There are not many practising doctors or dieticians who know anything other than the "sat fat is bad", "carbs are good" and "just cover it with insulin" mantras that persist, despite the evidence to the contrary.

Dieticians believe that starch is necessary for energy production in the body and that your brain will die if you don't eat at least 130g of dietary carbohydrate a day. They have not been taught that the liver makes as much as the brain requires even if you eat zero calories a day. This process is known as gluconeogenesis.

Diabetologists also believe that saturated fat causes insulin resistance. Saturated fat in the blood does indeed cause beta-cell dysfunction. But guess what? It is not dietary saturated fat that causes saturated fat in the blood[88]. The honours go to dietary carbohydrate, the very stuff that diabetics have been told to eat in huge quantities at every meal and then some. Dietary carbohydrate is turned into saturated fat by the liver. Dietary saturated fat is turned into unsaturated fat in the blood which is harmless.

Even diabetologists confuse benign dietary ketosis with the potentially life threatening diabetic ketoacidosis. They believe that the first can turn into the second unless you eat carbohydrates to stop it happening. Amazingly simplistic and amazingly wrong!

The sort of doctor likely to be attending to you, either as your GP or as your diabetologist, is also likely to be overloaded with work. They don't have the time to look further than their nose, and they trust the dieticians to give better advice to you about eating than they can. 'Thinking differently' isn't encouraged in the NHS and many GPs and diabetologists would rather wait for guidelines stating that low carbing is best for diabetes before they start promoting it for patients.

It is debatable if the culture in which NHS dieticians are raised is any better or worse than the culture in which doctors are raised, but there are only a few who will speak up about the dangers of carbohydrate overload such as the senior diabetes research fellow, Jacqui Troughton[89].

The supposed 'healthy' low-fat diet has enormous ramifications for the health services and economy of the developed world as obesity, type 2 diabetes and poorly controlled type one diabetes continue to rise exponentially.

At the same time, rationing of resources is going on due to the recession and medical workforce shortage, and the realisation that the costs of the obesity epidemic, among other things, is unsustainable. The cost of diabetes could, of course, be improved if PREVENTION of complications was given the attention it could be[90]. The cost of drugs, dialysis, surgeries and laser treatments could be cut if correct dietary principles were taught instead of the rubbish that is currently recommended for people with diabetes."

In the UK, there are some moves towards educating patients about their conditions and changing the culture of medicine towards a 'partnership' between the doctor and patient where clinical care decisions are evaluated, and responsibility for these are 'shared'. This approach is still in its infancy however and the "doctor" telling the "patient" what to do still rules.

Q. Can we rewind a bit? Are you saying saturated fats are healthy? I've always been told they are the foodstuff of the devil...

A. Dr Katharine Morrison: There was never any proof that saturated fats cause heart disease[91]. Unfortunately, the whole thing got off to a bad start when it was found that saturated fat does cause diseased arteries in... wait for it, RABBITS. It's an obvious point but bear in mind that rabbits are different from human beings, and their natural diet is all plant based.

The saturated fat/cholesterol theory then went off and was apparently confirmed when Ancel Keys, a USA researcher, produced his seven countries study in the 1950s, showing an association between dietary saturated fat and heart disease. He cherry picked his countries to show the connection.

When the data from all the 22 countries that were available at the time were examined, the correlation falls apart. For example, the Swiss eat an enormous amount of saturated fat yet they have low levels of heart disease. The Japanese eat very little saturated fat, and they have very low levels of heart disease, but higher numbers of haemorrhagic stroke[92].

Q. How do I eat when out and about?

A. Emma Baird: Actually, low-carb diets can be easy (much easier than a low-fat plan or having to count points and sins) when you are out and about, depending on how well organised you are willing to be.

Here are some general tips and ideas:

Many restaurants include their menus on their websites, so you can check these beforehand and work out what low-carb options there are.

Bistros and steak houses are obviously good choices for low-carb diets, but you can also ask restaurant staff can serve your dish without the chips and potatoes etc. Ask for additional veg or salad instead. Explain that you have blood sugar problems and need to avoid added sugars in your diet as a way of reinforcing your request.

In the main, you'll know to avoid the bread, potatoes and rice, as well as pasta dishes and pizza. Some sauces, though, may be loaded with sugar and/or flour. To avoid flour-based sauces, you can ask the restaurant for gluten-free options as most restaurants are aware of gluten-free requirements.

Many hotels often feature buffet options for breakfast and lunch. Choose sliced meats, fish, salads, vegetables, nuts, eggs and cheese and ignore anything with pastry, breads, potato salads and all of the sweet stuff at the end.

It might be an idea to carry round low-carb options which can double up as the odd emergency meal if you find yourself away from home and faced with only the sandwich option as a meal. A plastic box with some salad and dressing and a small packet of unsalted nuts, for example, or a package of sliced meat stored in a cool bag will keep you ticking over.

While most of us have grown up to accept sandwiches as the lunchtime option, the sandwich has only grown so hugely in popularity over the last 50 or so years. Funnily enough, so have levels of heart disease and type 2 diabetes... The natural lunchtime food? Perhaps not.

Q. Isn't constipation a problem with high-protein diets?

Emma Baird: High-protein diets some years ago featured very low amounts of vegetables and no fruit, which meant that some people may have experienced constipation as a result, but our recommendations for daily eating do include fruit and vegetables. You can eat plenty of salad leaves and green vegetables such as spinach, broccoli and kale to guard against constipation.

Because low-carbohydrate diets will make you wee a lot in the early days, it is important to ensure you are drinking plenty of fluids (and especially water) to help your bowels move everything along nicely.

Magnesium is a mineral that is often deficient in people with diabetes, and magnesium can help to "keep you regular" so it may be a good idea to start taking a magnesium supplement when you start on your low-carbohydrate diet to help with this. Two tablespoons of linseeds (buy them in your local health food store) taken daily with plenty of water can also assist.

Q. Can I be veggie and do a low-carbohydrate diet?

A. Emma Baird: What are your reasons for eating a vegetarian diet? If they are for health reasons, we hope we have given you enough grounds in the beginning chapters of this book as to why you should follow a low-carbohydrate diet and perhaps given you the reasons why eating meat and fish is good for you.

If you eat a vegetarian diet because of ethics, sourcing free-range and organic products can help you choose the animal products that have lived more in the way in that nature intended.

If you still feel strongly about not eating meat, or you don't eat meat because you do not like it, then you can still do a low-carbohydrate diet as a vegetarian.

You will probably have to aim for the upper carbohydrate limits of the low-carbohydrate diet in order to get enough variety and nutrients in your diet. Eating plenty of non-starchy vegetables, small amounts of beans and legumes, lots of nuts, eggs, cheese, Quorn, tofu (the non-genetically modified stuff) and fish if you choose to eat it, can make up a healthy diet.

The New Atkins for a New You diet book includes a section and recipes for vegetarians. You can also find plenty of low-carb recipes for vegetarians online.

Q. Talking of vegetarianism, what vegetables should I eat? I thought fruit was healthy, but you're telling me it isn't?

A. Emma Baird: We favour the non-starchy vegetables that grow above the ground as they have lower carb counts in them. Good vegetable choices include: artichokes, aubergines, baby sweet corn, bell peppers, broccoli, cabbage, celery, chicory, courgettes, cucumber, fennel, green beans, kale, mushrooms, rocket, salad leaves, spinach, spring onions and watercress.

Carrots and beetroot contain more carbohydrates than these vegetables, but if they are included grated in a pre-packed salad and in other small amounts, this is fine. Parsnips, potatoes, squashes and sweet potatoes all contain more carbohydrates than the above list of vegetables too, so should be weighed and measured before eating, with the appropriate insulin dose used to cover their consumption.

Fruit is healthy – but not in massive amounts. Ever heard the saying, the poison is in the dose? Many people over-do fruit in the belief that they are helping their health, but large amounts of fruit can contain a lot of carbohydrates and fast-acting sugar in the form of fructose. One to two portions of fruit a day should be your limit – and in fact, Dr Bernstein advocates that people with diabetes should not eat fruit at all[93].

As a rough guide (it depends on the size and ripeness of the fruit), here are the carbohydrate counts for popular fruits:

1. Apple, small apple (about 100g), 15g

2. Apricots (three small, whole ones), 12g

3. Banana, medium-sized, 20g (large ones can contain about 30g)

4. Blackberries (100g), 5g

5. Blueberries (100g), 5g

6. Cherries (100g), 16g

7. Grapes (100g), 18g

8. Orange, medium sized, 15g

9. Plums (two small ones), 12g

10. Raspberries (100g), 12g

11. Strawberries (100g), 7g

Strictly speaking, avocados and tomatoes are classed as fruits – but they do have less sugar than all of the above, and you can eat sliced tomatoes with your meals and add half an avocado to salads with only minimal carbohydrate addition. Tomato sauces are higher in carbohydrates because the tomatoes are more concentrated, but if you make your own, you can ensure there is no extra sugar added.

Dried fruit often used to be included in recipes for people with diabetes, but it is very high in sugar. Take 100g of currants, for instance. They contain 75g carbohydrates, compared to 18g for the equivalent of grapes. It is very easy to eat significant amounts of dried fruits because they are much smaller than their fresh equivalent so really you should avoid them or make them a very occasional treat.

Q. What about these low-carbohydrate products in my local health food store – the pasta, wraps and chocolate bars?

A. Emma Baird: Net carbs are the carbohydrates that remain in foods after the fibre content has been subtracted, so if we take broccoli as an example, with a carbohydrate content of 7g per 100g cooked, subtract the fibre content of 2g and you are left with 5g of net carbs. Fibre content is subtracted because this will not have an effect on your blood-sugar levels.

There is a proviso to this, however. No doubt you will have seen chocolate and other treat style sweet bars in health food shops and other supermarkets which refer to net carb totals – so a chocolate bar, for example, lists its carbohydrate content as 21g and yet states that only 2-3g of these are net carbs.

The reason for this claim is that the bars are usually sweetened with sugar alcohols (polyols). Sugar alcohols do have less of an effect on blood glucose levels than sugar and different people absorb them differently – so one person will absorb most of their carbohydrate content, while another person's body will not. If you choose to eat these bars and other products marketed as high-carbohydrate, it would be wise to check your blood sugar levels an hour after eating.

Personally, I find that I need to take insulin with these so-called low-carbohydrate chocolate bars, and the amount of insulin I need is an amount to cover the total carbohydrate count minus the fibre (not the polyols), which is a higher amount than the net carbs stated on the packet.

One final thing – one of the issues with polyols is that they can have a laxative effect and consuming them in large quantities can cause bloating, flatulence and diarrhoea. Kind of off-putting, hmm?

Q. I'm female; does that make it harder to control my blood sugar?

A. Dr Katharine Morrison: Male and female children have the same issues around blood sugar till around the age of 10 when pubertal changes in girls raise insulin resistance and it all starts to go a bit pear shaped.

Girls reach peak insulin resistance around 12-13 and have very difficult-to-manage blood sugars due to this, and due to the hormonal fluctuations around their menstrual cycles. Also, teenage girls tend to fall out with their main care giver, their mother, more often than boys do, again making blood sugar control for girls more difficult.

Girls tend to have more carbohydrate craving than boys and tend to want to fit in more with other girls. This can mean that they don't want to eat differently from their friends and this often means either eating cakes, biscuits, sweets and chocolates or at the other end of the scale doing various calorie controlled diets that always seem to start on Mondays.

In my experience, women find sticking to low carb diets harder than men, and they lose weight at a much slower pace than men. Young men often keep up sports or recreational football whereas girls often do no sports once they stop doing these things at school. As everyone knows, weight gain is a common feature of pregnancy, and this weight may not be fully lost after each pregnancy.

For type 1 women, stringent blood sugar control during pregnancy is of particular importance. You would think that women get a break once the menopause occurs, but women get more insulin resistant, and although they no longer have hormonal fluctuations, they do need to keep dietary carbs down and exercise up to maintain a favourable weight and degree of fitness.

All in all, it is in my opinion much harder being a diabetic woman than being a diabetic man.

Emma Baird: Me too (last time I looked). Seriously though, like many type 1 female diabetics, I notice changes in my blood sugar levels in the week before my period is due. This is because I experience insulin resistance in that time, meaning that my body needs more insulin to cope with the hormonal changes going on in my body.

Q. I've suddenly got a flat stomach. What's happening to me?

A. Emma Baird: Finally, we get to the lovely bits! A flat, or flatter stomach is one of the common side effects of a low-carbohydrate diet. Ever heard the saying, abs are made in the kitchen? A common misconception is that visible abdominal muscles, and a flat stomach is due to thousands of sit up, crunches or any other stomach exercise you see promoted by some kind of trendy fitness professional.

However, a low-carbohydrate diet will force the body into choosing fat and not sugar as its preferred energy source. When you eat carbohydrates, this often forces the body to store more water. As you first start out on a low-carbohydrate diet, the body will start to release all of that stored water (in other words you will spend the first few days of a low-carbohydrate diet peeing) which will result in dramatic weight loss. This will even out as the body adjusts.

Excess carbohydrates in the diet tend to result in bigger and fatter stomachs because the excess sugar is stored as fat around the middle because the body cannot use it effectively.

The other welcome side effects you may experience can include:

Better sleep (because your body isn't dealing with fluctuating blood sugar levels during the day and night)

Better energy levels during the day – again because your body isn't experiencing varying sugar levels

Decrease in appetite – higher protein, high-fat and low-carbohydrate diets tend to reduce the appetite naturally because your sugar levels are stable. If you choose to eat eggs in the morning, for example, you will probably notice that you do not get hungry until lunch time or later. If you are used to eating cereal and/or toast in the morning, you are probably familiar with the feeling of hunger, and the need to snack come 11am.

Better skin – again, normal blood sugar levels will improve your skin, and you can wave goodbye to rashes, redness and boils.

Better happiness levels – guess what? When you aren't fighting tiredness because you are battling fluctuating blood sugar levels, this gives you increased energy and a better sense of well-being. And who doesn't want to be happier?

Q. Can I drink alcohol on a low-carb diet?

Yes, you can, but only very lightly. Type 2s may stick with government guidelines. For men and women, this is 2-3 units a day with two alcohol-free days a week.

Alcohol contains calories that you probably don't need. It also tends to increase your appetite and reduce your willpower. Positive effects are that it does reduce stress for some people and there are some cardiovascular benefits from drinking low amounts of red wine compared to drinking nothing at all. This amount is low, however, and is only half a glass a day! Total mortality rises in women after only 4 units of alcohol a week.

Here are some calories for alcoholic drinks:

1. Beer 500ml 160
2. Sweet cider 500mls 210
3. Gin, Vodka 25mls 56
4. Bailey's Irish Cream 25mls 80
5. Red wine 175mls 119
6. Dry white wine 116

If you use insulin, there are more important issues than calories to consider.

When you are eating less than 130g of carb a day, your liver will be required to make up to this amount of glucose as you will no longer be obtaining it from your food. There is usually no problem at all with this.

However, if you consume a lot of alcohol you will prevent your liver from making glucose, and you may get severe hypoglycaemia. Therefore, you should only drink if you are eating something along with it and stick to the sensible drinking limits at all times. Whatever alcohol you may have got away with on a high carb diet, you might not on a low carb diet, particularly if you are going below 50g of carb a day.

Q. What are the best methods of contraception to use with diabetes?

Dr Katharine Morrison: There are many different methods of contraception, and individual circumstances will dictate which are the best options for you. Because foetal abnormalities are a considerable risk with high blood sugars, it is always best to plan a pregnancy when you have had a chance to get blood sugars and any complications dealt with. Effective contraception is, therefore, even more important for diabetic women.

If you are overweight, this could be worsened particularly by the contraceptive injection Depo-Provera. Weight can increase with other hormonal methods (for example, the combined oral contraceptive pill, the Mirena coil and progestogen implant and the progestogen only pill), but are not as marked.

Completely non-hormonal methods of contraception include the copper coil and condoms. Coils do not prevent ectopic pregnancies.

Copper coils increase the amount of menstrual flow up to about three times that of usual so are not suitable if you have heavy periods or period pains to start with. Condoms are notoriously unreliable and, if you use baby oil as a lubricant, this will perish the rubber. Condoms should be used with water-based lubricants. They can reduce the risk of contracting sexually transmitted diseases when used correctly.

If you are an insulin-using diabetic, it can really help if you can get rid of the peaks and troughs of blood sugar variation caused by menstrual cycles. Methods that provide contraception but don't avoid the peaks and troughs would be to use the combined oral contraceptive pill taken in the traditional (but unnecessary) 21 days on, 7 days off pattern, condoms on their own, and the copper coil.

Useful methods to even out hormonal imbalances are: Mirena coil or Cerazette, the most efficient progestogen only pill. Loestrin 20 or other 20 micrograms combined contraceptive pill taken every day without a break will also lead to a stable hormonal status. If you do have a bleed, stop the pill for four days and then resume.

Depo-Provera can also be used to stabilise the hormonal state, but it does increase insulin resistance and therefore weight to at least some extent. Implants also work well for this, but often result in bleeding during the first six months of use. They do last for three years though.

If you have acne, Depo-Provera would be a method to avoid as it tends to worsen the condition. Suitable methods would be "friendly" progestogen/oestrogen preparations such as Mercilon and Marvelon.

If you smoke or have complications of diabetes, you are best to stay away from methods of contraception that contain oestrogen as this increases arterial risk to some extent. This would be all combined oral contraceptive pills or vaginal rings. Useful techniques would be all of the progestogen pills, implants and copper and Mirena coils.

If you have any particular high risk of osteoporosis such as having an eating disorder, rheumatoid arthritis, have absent periods for medical reasons you are best to avoid Depo-Provera for any long length of time. Other methods that may be more suitable are oestrogen containing contraceptives.

As you can see, there are choices and compromises about all the methods. You can be guided by your GP, and if you have a particularly challenging issue that needs to be addressed, you can be referred to a contraceptive clinic in your area. Often you simply self-refer.

The Family Planning Association website has a lot of information about all methods of contraception. They have a "my contraception" tool that gives you individualised advice based on your clinical history and preferences[94].

Q. What should I do if I am planning a pregnancy?

Dr Katharine Morrison: If you are planning a pregnancy you should speak to your GP and get referred to a specialist clinic that has input from a consultant obstetrician and a consultant diabetologist who are interested and experienced in the care of pregnant women with diabetes.

They will want to encourage you to get your blood sugars as tight as possible. This is certainly under an HbA1c of 7% and ideally under 6%. The tightest levels of control are only possible on a low carb diet. Dr Jovanovich, who is the foremost specialist in this subject, advises a diet of no more than 90g -120g of carb a day. This has recently been recommended for all diabetics by the American Association of Clinical Endocrinologists[95].

Their 2013 guideline advises that half of the carbohydrate consumed should be low starch vegetables and the remainder may be fruit or starch. This could mean that at each meal you may have, in addition to two or three portions of low starch vegetables, one tiny portion of bread/potatoes/rice etc. or one moderate piece of fruit.

The clinic can arrange for insulin pumps, carb counting lessons, ophthalmic review and whatever other input is necessary.

You will also need to take folic acid 5mg daily. This is available on prescription from your GP.

Q. Can I follow a low carb diet during pregnancy?

Yes. In fact, it is almost impossible to get HbA1cs below 6.0 % without risk of severe hypoglycaemia unless you do. This is the optimal level of blood sugar control for pregnancy. Dr Lois Jovanovich and Dr Richard Bernstein manage their diabetic patients with low carb diets of varying degrees of carbohydrate intake ranging from 30 to 135g per day.

Ideally, you would have an HbA1c under 6.0% for two months before conception. You may need to have an insulin pump to control basal insulin levels, particularly if you have a prominent dawn phenomenon, raising morning blood sugars. A recent USA study found that average HbA1c in pregnant women, not using low carb diets, was 8.1% and this dropped to 7.5% for those on insulin pumps. As you can see, many women do not manage to obtain ideal blood sugar control, and you should do everything you can to reduce blood sugars and minimise hypos well before conception if at all possible.

It is worth noting that you may get urinary ketones quite often on a low carb diet. When in small amounts as occurs with dietary ketosis, they do not indicate or lead to diabetic ketoacidosis. Ketone production due to fat metabolism products on a low carb diet is associated with normal blood sugars and reduced hypoglycaemia and is caused by a relative lack in dietary carbohydrate.

If you increase dietary carbohydrate, it goes away. Diabetic ketoacidosis is caused by a relative lack of insulin and is often precipitated by infection of some kind. Blood sugars are very high and get a lot worse with increasing dietary carbohydrate.

Q. What is the best way to prevent low blood sugars when you exercise?

Dr Katharine Morrison: The two primary methods to avoid low blood sugars are to cut the insulin you inject or eat more carbohydrate, or a mixture of both if you are exercising vigorously or for an extended period of time.

What you choose to do will depend on whether you want to lose weight or not.

Exercise burns a lot fewer calories than it often feels like at the time. An hour's walk for instance only burns round about 100 calories. This is as much as a fried egg's worth. Do NOT believe what the machines in the gym tell you – this information is inaccurate, and the fitness industry is very disingenuous about calorie burn as it suits the industry to promote the message that exercise will make you lose weight.

Insulin users are best to exercise at the same time each day if they possibly can. This way, they can adjust their basal (background insulin) or meal insulins around the exercise.

You can either take less insulin for a meal than you really need if you are going for a walk soon after, or give yourself something extra to eat, for example, a dessert, a piece of fruit, or extra starch at that meal. If you are going outside the house to exercise, always carry extra food, glucose tablets or Lucozade with you.

When diabetics are running high blood sugars all the time, as in NHS management, they don't necessarily get hypos when doing more activity than they are used to. When you start to run your blood sugars much nearer normal, that is around 4.6mmol/l (82mg), you will notice that extra activity will give you lower blood sugars.

If your blood sugar management is improving to the tighter levels we recommend, remember to factor this into your day. For those who are keen to lose weight the thing to do is to cut the insulin for that time of day and for several hours later.

If you are thin or of normal weight, you have the option to eat more carbohydrate.

Emma Baird: A word of warning! If your blood sugar is over 11mmol/l (198mg) before exercising, you will find exercise very difficult indeed. This is because the body sends even more glucose into the blood to cope with the tiredness. Either choose to exercise a different day when you are feeling better, or take a little bit of insulin (half the usual dose you need to correct) and ensure that you test your blood sugar during and after exercise.

Q. I use insulin. What do I do if I feel ill?

Diabetics who use insulin need to be particularly vigilant when it comes to acute illness.

The main problem is that any infection or any potentially dehydrating illness such as vomiting or severe diarrhoea can lead to diabetic ketoacidosis. You will, therefore, do what anyone else would do for any particular illness, BUT in general, you would contact your health care provider much earlier in the course of the illness, AND you would start hyper-vigilant blood sugar/ketone monitoring every 2 and a half hours instead of every 5 hours.

To deal with the diabetic issues with illness efficiently and effectively, I highly recommend that insulin users buy Dr Richard Bernstein's Diabetes Solutions. This book has the best advice for dealing with acute illness, as well as many other things that I know about. There is little point in stumbling over it for the first time when you are ill, however. It is important that you, family and friends have read and understood the advice given ahead of time. If a diabetic lives away from home, e.g. at university, it is worth having a copy of the book at both sites.

Q. Are dietary supplements useful or are they just a waste of money?

Dr Katharine Morrison: Some dietary supplements are worthwhile. The problem is that these substances have not been subjected to the same rigorous evaluation as most drugs have. Many supplements that claim to have "anti-ageing" actions, for instance, but no randomised controlled trial has ever been done on them.

The ones that I think are worthwhile are vitamin D3 and magnesium and, for particular groups, omega 3 fatty acids, vitamin B compound, glucosamine and chondroitin and a multivitamin (without iron).

I have tested about 200 patients in my practice area (the west coast of Scotland; an area which does not get much sunlight) and so far have found that 15 had undetectable levels of vitamin D. Of the others 90% had severe deficiency with a level of around 25 and 10% had levels around 50.

You need to have levels of more than 50 to prevent bone disease and 160 to obtain the full benefits of vitamin D supplementation. Vitamin D receptors are present in most cells of the body and these cells function best when they receive adequate vitamin D. This is why vitamin D deficiency causes such a wide variety of problems and supplementation has such immense benefits.

Problems of deficiency include rickets, osteoporosis, psoriasis, higher rates of multiple sclerosis, higher rates of cancers including breast, colorectal and prostate cancers, reduced insulin sensitivity, neurological disorders, gingivitis, and infections.

Vitamin D3 is available online from amazon.co.uk for only £8 for a year's supply including postage. I used to test before advising supplements but because almost everyone is deficient in Scotland and blood test rationing to once a year has come in, what I advise is taking 1,000 iu daily of Vitamin D3 daily for every 30 pounds body weight and then getting a blood sample taken after three months. You can take the drug daily or weekly. If your blood level is under 160 then up the amount and test in another year. If your level is over 200, then cut back and check in another year.

Magnesium deficiency is said to be widespread because there is not enough of it in the soil. Magnesium is essential for bone health, but also because it relaxes smooth muscle. The smooth muscle that lines your arteries is also affected by this and magnesium can, therefore, help people who have hypertension. Magnesium has also been found to improve insulin sensitivity. The dose is 400-800mg a day. Only use the higher dose range if you have hypertension or arterial disease. When you buy a supplement for the first time, buy it in a small quantity because some preparations have a marked laxative effect. Once you have something that suits you, you can buy it in greater amounts. You can also buy Epsom salts which are high in magnesium and add them to your bath water.

Omega 3 fatty acids are present in seafood and fish, particularly oily fish. If you don't like eating these perhaps an omega 3 fatty acid capsule a day 500-1000mg would be a good idea. These oils are said to improve the elasticity of cell walls. In randomised controlled trials they were found to reduce cardiac arrhythmias.

Vitamin B compound can be especially useful for avoiding midge and mosquito bites. It makes your sweat less attractive to biting insects. If you have a hard time with these wee beasties on your outdoor walking and exercise sessions, then you could try these and see what happens. They are very cheap and widely available. Be warned: they do turn your urine bright yellow. Eating garlic also works well to deter these annoying wee beasties.

Glucosamine and Chondroitin supplements help some people with knee arthritis. If you take the tablets in full dosage for two months and they have not improved your knees, then they are unlikely to work for you.

A multi vitamin (without iron) may be helpful for those who do not eat much in the way of vegetables and fruit on the one hand and meat on the other. In Scotland, many people don't eat anything like three vegetables and two pieces of fruit daily as recommended, so if you can't stand the green stuff then perhaps a multi-vitamin would be a good idea. [It's a better idea to make yourself like fruit and vegetables.]

If you eat lots of vegetables and fruit, but avoid meat or eat very little of it, then you may not be getting enough vitamin B12 and perhaps other B vitamins. A multi vitamin may be helpful for you.

The reason why most people should avoid iron is that it acts as an oxidant. When there is too much of it in the body iron contributes to atherosclerosis, tissue ageing and cancer. Diabetics have enough of a problem with high blood sugars doing the same thing, never mind adding to the problem with iron. The groups that need to avoid excess iron are men over the age of 30 and non-menstruating women and anyone who has been diagnosed with haemochromatosis or other iron storage conditions. If you do have iron deficiency anaemia for whatever reason, then you can take a multi vitamin with added iron, but you may do better to eat plenty of red meat, drink a small amount of fruit juice or take a vitamin C supplement with your meals and avoid tea or coffee with your meals.

Q. How do I get what needs to be done at my diabetes checks?

Most doctors in General Practice and Hospital medicine have check lists of what they want to achieve in a consultation with a patient. Often these are purely procedural and do not necessarily have particular relevance to that patient at that time. Doctors tend to be very rushed and constrained by time, and it is easy to intend to ask about something that is bothering you, but find that it has slipped from your mind when you walk out of the consultation.

It is helpful for the doctor or nurse to have in writing exactly what issues you need to be addressed at the start of the discussion. This way they can hopefully deal with your problem. The patient concerns form in the appendix is a useful thing to photocopy and use. It was designed by Martha Funnell who is a diabetes nurse and educator in the USA who has done a lot of research about patient-health professional communication.

The three-day food diary/blood sugar sheets that are available online in the appendix are constructive for yourself and your doctor in finding out what is going right and what is not optimal about your blood-sugar control. It can be used to determine whether you have the dawn phenomenon or not, whether your basal insulin needs increased or not, and what your meal/carb sensitivity ratios are. If you are new to low carbing, it can be used to practice carb counting, and you can see if your pancreas can cope with whatever glucose load you have set your mind on.

Some clinics give patients their results so that they can keep a personal tab on their weight, BMI, waist circumference, HbA1, blood pressure, lipid tests, urinary protein tests, foot checks and eye checks. The trend in these is always helpful for you and your doctor to have.

Bring an up to date list of your medication and insulin types and doses. The medical history sheet can be used for this and for hospital admissions.

Q. I am going into hospital for an operation. What preparations should I make?

When you have a date to go into hospital for a planned procedure a person with diabetes has the same sort of thing as everyone else has to do…and then some more.

You need to arrange for someone to look after your house and any animals. You need to bring in nightwear and usually also daywear such as a track suit and slippers. You need the usual dressing gown, underwear, socks, spectacles, books, money, change, phone and charger. Wet wipes, dental care, hair care, face and body care products and deodorant are necessary. You may also need a tin opener, bottles of water, cans of food and individual packs of fruit in juice may come in useful. Your own towels and even sheet or two may be necessary. You may need a set of cutlery, salt and pepper.

It is doubtful that the hospital will offer a low carb diet for diabetics or anyone else. Hospitals budget around less than 0.5 percent of the NHS budget on food and drink. The food is usually very high in starchy carbohydrate, low in protein and high in polyunsaturated fats because firstly they are cheap and secondly, they are approved of as being "healthy" by government agencies such as the Food Standards Agency.

Good blood sugar management is critical at any time, but particularly if you are going to be having an operation or are at risk of getting an infection. Believe me, just being in a hospital puts you at risk of infection. It is therefore important to stress, preferably before you go in, that you will be choosing, not from the "diabetic" section of the meal plan but from the "normal" section of the meal plan and that you will be selecting the portion sizes that suit you.

By doing this, you will probably be able to have some sort of protein and vegetable meal at lunch and dinner. Breakfast has become a toast and cereal fest at most hospitals with barely an egg in sight. If you can get a cooked breakfast, then do your best with it. It is better to be prepared and bring in low carb baking that can be kept in plastic boxes and have a tin opener and some tins of salmon, tuna or corned beef. You can get individual containers of fruit in juice which may come in handy.

I, Katharine, have been an inpatient several times and have used every single item that I have mentioned during at least one admission because the hospital did not provide it. If you have any items left, you can give them away to your grateful ward mates when you leave.

For insulin users, it is essential that you take in your blood sugar testing kit, insulin pens, pump and spare items that you think you may need. Keep them beside you, although spare insulin may be stored in the ward fridge.

If you are at all able to do so, it is far preferable that you check your own blood sugars, and give your own insulin, in the dose that you know suits you. If your doses need to be altered the doctor or nurse should be able to give you a reasonable reason why. Don't just take their word for it that they know what they are doing. Medication errors are widespread in hospitals. It can be lethal if the wrong dose or type of insulin is given.

If you are in an open ward tell your fellow patients that you are diabetic and tell them how to recognise a hypo and what to do about it. This would usually involve, asking you to check your blood sugar and getting a nurse.

When you are admitted to hospital, you will be "clerked in" by a junior hospital doctor and nurse and anyone else involved in your treatment. This means asking you everything about yourself by several different people, several different times. It can be beneficial if you have filled in the information in medical history sheet, particularly if this is typewritten, and you have at least two copies of it. This way you can save them time and you, aggravation. Medication errors also tend to be reduced.

When you go into hospital, your primary task should be on staying safe and getting better. It is helpful to organise one primary source of contact, a close friend or relative, who will contact your other friends to deal with household matters and a visit rota.

If they will look after animals, plants, the mail, put the bins out on the right day, and open and shut curtains it is a great help. If they remove things that will go off from the fridge and empty the bins when you go in, and put the heating back on, and put a supply of useful perishable items in your fridge for when you get back, it can make a great deal of difference to your recovery.

And finally... No more questions but a little learning point. Years ago, many of us took what doctors and other medical professionals said as gospel. If a physician told you to do so and so, you tended to do it without question. There is no doubt that medical training and clinical experience are very worthwhile and it produces experts in health. However, what your doctor or dietician tells you is not always based on the most up to date information and findings. Let's look at this example...

Dr Katharine Morrison:

"One example of the culture of medical school that I recall is when my biochemistry lab partner and I, along with several other students, did not get the 'right' results from an experiment. We were told by post grad students who were supervising us that they would lock the lab door and we wouldn't get out until we had rubbed out all our 'wrong' results with therefore the 'wrong' answer and replaced them with some 'right' results and therefore the 'right' answer.

Although I had been encouraged to think about sources of experimental error at school this idea had still to catch on at university medical school. "Education" continued in this vein into the clinical years where "doing it the right way" was enforced. Original thought and doing anything differently, no matter how beneficial, were not tolerated and usually resulted in derision. I remember the first time the idea that peptic ulcers were caused by a bacteria (a true discovery that revolutionised the outlook for these patients) was presented to a lecture room full of doctors. You may have expected curiosity.... but what you got were denial, mirth and outright hostility.

It is particularly ironic that the academic qualifications to get into medical school are spectacularly high when the entire culture of medicine is geared to bullying these bright, idealistic young people into doing whatever they are told regardless of scientific validity".

CHAPTER 9

MACRONUTRIENTS, MICRONUTRIENTS AND SAMPLE MENU PLANS

In this chapter, we are going to take a look at some sample menu plans you can use to help you get used to low-carb eating, but before we start, let's look at macro nutrients and micro nutrients.

PROTEIN

Macro nutrients are protein, carbohydrates and fat. Let's start with protein. If you consult the plates so revered by the UK's National Health Service and the USA Department of Agriculture, these two institutions recommend that around 15% of your calories should come from protein. We think that level is too low and that 20-30% is a better number to aim for.

A good way to establish how much protein is necessary for you is to take your ideal weight in kilograms and divide it by six.[96] This gives the minimum amount of dietary protein to maintain your muscle mass. Thus, a 60kg woman would need 10oz (or about 285g)[97] of lean protein a day rather than the 5.5oz (155g) suggested by the USDA food pyramid. A woman may eat more than this, say 15oz (425g) or even up to 20oz (560g). A 70kg man would need 11.6oz (329g) as a minimum.

Instead of having protein as a minor part of a starch-based meal, you are better to be eating a meal that is based around protein. The form that it takes will be up to you. Fish, white meat, eggs and nuts are good for everyone. Red meats are beneficial for growing children and menstruating women. For men over 30 years of age and post-menopausal women, they might be better to limit red meat to four times a week.[98]

The amount of fat that the meat may contain is irrelevant. Enjoy it. This news may come as a surprise to you, especially if you have spent years following a low-fat/ high carb diet where you are always told to cut the fat off meat and skip treats such as crispy chicken skin. So, here is why it is important to eat fat. Natural sources of fat such as fatty cuts of meat, egg yolks, fish, nuts, avocados and olives contain vitamins and can help protect the body against heart disease.[99] Fat in the diet blunts blood sugar spikes[100] and also does not need to be covered by insulin.

Red meat should be limited in amount for adult men and women who have stopped menstruating. This is because the iron in red meat is particularly easily absorbed by the gut. Absorption of iron is enhanced by alcohol, vitamin C, fruit juice, and sugar and reduced by tea, coffee and eggs. If accumulated in excessive amounts it acts as an oxidiser and can cause inflammation in the body. The increased iron problem is probably the cause for the association between red meat and cancer[101].

Processed meats such as bacon, sausages and chorizo are also associated with increased rates of bowel cancer so should also be limited in the diet.

Stick to meat which closely resembles what you would have caught in the wild as a hunter-gatherer – and if you can eat meat that has come from grass-fed animals, all the better.

As you will have noted from the earlier chapters about the medications needed for meals, protein if eaten in any quantity over 3oz (75g) in a meal will need to be covered with insulin. It does increase blood sugar in diabetics and does so over a long length of time. A steak, for instance, can raise the blood sugar for up to 10 hours.

Regular acting insulin, which lasts for five hours but has a tail of eight hours, is a good insulin to use to cover protein meals. If you take insulin, the formula you can use is two units of regular insulin to cover 3oz (75g), or a deck of cards size of the steak[102], for example.

Humulin S and Hypurin Soluble. Cartridges are available in the UK for this purpose (they are 'regular' insulins). In the USA, you can use Humulin S cartridges or Actrapid vials since pork insulins are difficult to get there.

Adequate protein is necessary to limit muscle wasting which is common as people age.

In fact, bodies start to lose muscle mass at the relatively young age of 25, with an average loss of 0.5-1% a year from that age.

Some down sides to eating protein are that this macro nutrient is expensive, tends to spoil quickly, and eating enough protein can be a challenge for non-meat eaters. You will find that you need to plan meals in advance, shop more frequently for fresh ingredients and that you may enjoy it more if you improve and diversify your cooking skills.

Beans and legumes such as lentils are also often included in "protein" source information. The problem with these foods is that they also tend to be high in carbohydrate. They are by no means the worst foods to eat, but the carbohydrate needs to be considered. These foods can also cause some people a lot of wind because they contain fermenting sugars and they have come in from criticism because they may inhibit the absorption of minerals, such as magnesium and calcium, from the gut. On the other hand, they also inhibit iron absorption which in some cases can be a good thing.

Good advice is to eat beans and legumes in small amounts and make them an adjunct to your protein-containing meal rather than the main focus. This can be done by, for example, having some kidney beans in your chilli con carne, by adding vegetables such as carrots and celery to your lentil soup or by having one or two tablespoons of baked beans with your bacon, eggs and tomato rather than having a full can of them.

The Filling Power of Protein

Adequate protein in the diet is a very useful as a tool to fill you up. You would generally divide your protein so that you have some at every meal.

Diabetics who use insulin are much better off having three meals a day rather than snacking between meals – and having enough protein in your meals can help to fill you up so that you do not need to snack.

If you do not snack, then the insulin you have used to cover that meal will be almost finished before the next meal. If you eat between meals, you need to give yourself another injection of insulin, and you end up stacking one meal's insulin on top of another. In turn, this makes it impossible to know how much insulin is still active before the next meal.

FATS

Ah, fat... This particular macro nutrient has been demonised for years – and still continues to be. Walk into any supermarket, and there will be shelves groaning with products marked low or reduced fat, while the mainstream dieting industry continues to pick out fat as the big no-no.

(And meanwhile, food manufacturers condone the addition of sugar or low-fat products which resemble nothing that you find in nature).

Choosing to eat a low-carbohydrate eating plan means eating plenty of natural, healthy fats – which is great news because such fats can make your food taste really great and they are filling. Think about it – what would you rather have; a fresh salad dressed with a too sharp and sugary-tasting, low-fat dressing[103], or a fresh salad dressed with a tablespoon of olive oil, balsamic vinegar and sea salt?

Naturally, saturated fat such as those from butter and coconut oil is stable at higher temperatures than omega three and omega six oils and are ideal for cooking and baking[104]. They provide some benefits and do no harm to the body if not eaten to caloric excess. Let's term these oils neutral.

Omega six fats found in vegetable and seed oils and margarines are cheap, widely available and are used extensively in processed foods. They produce inflammation in the body and are associated with increased rates of diabetes, atherosclerosis and cancers[105]. They are harmful and best avoided.

Artificial trans- fats are also damaging to the body and are best avoided.[106] Again, if you cut out processed foods and refined carbohydrates from your diet, then you will naturally be avoiding artificial trans- fats. The naturally occurring trans- fats, such as conjugated linoleic acid, by contrast, are beneficial[107]. Conjugated linoleic acid is found mainly in beef and dairy products.

Oils are scarcely mentioned in the UK guideline. They are referred to in the USA food pyramid, but the wrong emphasis has been put on them. Omega 3 fats from seafood and extra virgin olive oil and flaxseed oil are known to improve cardiovascular health[108]. They can go rancid fast and should not be used for deep frying. They can be eaten in large quantities, but taste and expense tend to limit their use. These oils are beneficial.

TOO SALTY OR NOT?

There is some dubiety about whether a high salt intake is a problem or not.

Most conventional health organisations recommend lowering salt intakes, primarily because of its perceived effect on blood pressure.

In the western diet, about 75-90% of the salt that most people eat comes from its addition to processed food. Salt can help preserve food and, when it is added, there is sometimes a need for less sugar to be added for taste. Common sources of high-salt containing foods include bread, breakfast cereals, snack foods, tinned soups, packet sauces, and tinned meat and fish.

In contrast, the backbone of a healthy menu for diabetics is fresh, unprocessed food. You will find that your salt intake falls naturally with a low carbohydrate, adequate protein, and high-fat diet.

Indeed, in the early phases of a strict, low-carb diet you may have to add extra salt to your food to avoid "induction flu"[109]. This is partly due to the decreased amount taken in from the lack of bread and other processed foods and partly due to the increased excretion of salt, through urination, on a low-carb diet.

CARBOHYDRATES

We've looked at protein and fats, so that leaves carbohydrates. As previously discussed, you may have been taught to make the basis of your diet for diabetes around whole grain carbohydrates, choosing wholemeal bread, wholemeal pasta, brown rice and baked, boiled or mashed potatoes, and having the very occasional "treat" of sweets, cakes or chocolates, crisps and other high-fat, high carbohydrate items.

We want you to re-think your carbohydrates. Instead of thinking of them in terms of bread, rice, potatoes and pasta, consider them as vegetables and fruit. According to the "health" plates, we looked at earlier, fruit and vegetables are meant to make up about a third of your calories. There is no problem with this recommendation, except to say that sweet fruit is not in the same category as non-starchy vegetables when it comes to blood sugar control for diabetics. Rather than thinking "fruit and veg", make it "veg and SOME fruit".

The best vegetables for diabetics are vegetables that grow above the ground. Eat as many as you want and douse them generously with butter or extra virgin olive oil. This greatly enhances the taste, and the extra fat provides calories and increases absorption of the vitamins and minerals in the vegetables.

Fruit such as tomatoes, peppers and avocados are not particularly high in carbohydrate and can be treated much the same as low starch vegetables. Avocados are quite fatty with a high amount of unsaturated natural oils that have health benefits in that they are a natural anti-inflammatory food.

Vegetables such as parsnips, sweet potatoes, squashes, beetroot and potatoes are very starchy and can add to your total carbohydrate load if they are eaten in any quantity. Carrots and turnip also grow below ground, but can usually be eaten in moderate amounts particularly as part of a meal such as with a meat stew or grated in a salad and dressed with olive oil.

Temperate fruit such as apples and pears have around 15-20g of carbohydrate per piece, depending on their size and type. They can be eaten at the end of a meal without raising blood sugars too much, and the blood sugar spike can be blunted with the addition of cream or cheese.

Berries and melon are overall quite low in their effects on blood sugar and can be eaten in moderate amounts without problems. A handful of berries or a slice of cantaloupe melon will have about 7.5g of carbohydrate in them.

Tropical fruit such as pineapples, bananas and mangoes have more sugar in them than the berries and more temperate fruit. An average sized banana has 30g of carbohydrate in it. A portion size would be about half of a banana. These fruits can be eaten, but you will need to pay more attention to portion sizes as bananas can vary significantly in size and it can be easy to eat large amounts of grapes. They may be useful items to eat to cover exercise or can be eaten in small portions after a protein/fat/vegetable meal.

Fruit juice and smoothies have little place in a diet that is helpful for diabetics. They are very high in sugar and often calories. They are easy to drink in quantity and are best avoided. Tomato juice is relatively low in carbohydrate compared to orange juice, so consider this if you are looking for a different soft drink.

Tinned fruit may be found with syrup or fruit juice. Use the fruit juice version and drain off the juice before eating.

Frozen fruit and vegetables can be as good nutritionally as fresh. They can be eaten all year round, and you only need to defrost the quantity you intend to eat.

MILK AND DAIRY

Government-recommended diets give almost as much attention to milk and dairy as they give to protein. Milk, yoghurt and cheese can provide a healthy source of protein and fats, but its place in health is controversial, and many people can't eat dairy products because of intolerance.

A recommendation of three cups of dairy a day or equivalent is advised, but if you chose to take your milk and dairy recommendation as milk, then three servings would stack up to 30g of carbohydrate.

More concentrated protein and healthy fats can be obtained from other food sources without the carbohydrates, such as yoghurt or cheese, but there are various problems with eating a lot of dairy apart from the carbohydrate issues.

Some people, especially those of Asian ancestry, are intolerant of dairy products. It is the second most prevalent food allergen after wheat. There are also ethical reasons for avoiding dairy products. To sustain milk production, cows are impregnated every year and can be milked intensively – on some large-scale farms this can happen up to three times a day. Also, most calves are not reared alongside their mothers. Some calves are factory farmed for their meat in narrow stalls – called the Dutch crate system.

Matters would be improved for these calves if the populace in the UK ate more home-grown pink veal. Meanwhile, if you are conscious of animal welfare, it does make sense to cut down the amount of milk we drink. This does tend to happen on a low carb diet as fewer milky drinks are consumed, and breakfast cereals aren't usually eaten. Meanwhile for those tolerant of dairy products, on a low-carbohydrate diet, you can eat cheese, cream and butter. Just as with protein sources, we recommend organic dairy products or those which come from grass-fed sources.

OUR EXPERIENCES

Dr Morrison – From my own observations and experiments, I have found that I maintain a weight of 9st 5lbs (131lbs) on a caloric intake of 2,150 calories. I am 5ft 5.5 ins. I eat 23% of my calories from protein, 35-80g carbs and the rest made up of fat.

Just as an example of how this might work when out and about, take a buffet situation. When presented with a buffet, I tend to eat about double the amount of meat/fish or eggs than those people who also eat the more usual amounts of starch. I then have some salad or prepared vegetables, followed by cheese and fruit.

Emma – I am 5ft 2" and I shoot for a weight of about 8st 10lbs (122lbs) and I aim for 20% protein, 50-60g carbs (15%) and the rest from fat.

One of the pieces of advice that I think really works for people who eat a low-carb diet is for you to cease thinking of certain foods as 'breakfast' or 'lunch' items. The concept of cereal for breakfast or sandwiches for lunch is a marketing idea backed up by billions of pounds. Eating protein-based breakfasts and lunches will leave you feeling much more satisfied anyway.

SAMPLE MENU PLANS

What are your personal targets? These may change over time. Here, we are going to outline what you should eat depending on these targets. We'll give you a sample week plan for people wanting to eat very low-carbohydrate (under 50g) and one for people who want to aim for the more moderate 50-90g carbs a day.

If you wish to eat more carbohydrates and you have worked out how you can manage your medication to allow you to do so, then we suggest you individually add 10-15g of carbohydrates to each of the meals in the moderate menu plan suggestions. Using your newly-acquired knowledge of food and its carbohydrate content, you can choose to add a slice of bread, some potatoes, an amount of rice, some fruit, beans or legumes and other choices to your diet.

Where we have specified values, you need to measure these foods so that you know how many carbohydrates you are eating and how much medication you need. For protein, remember the regular insulin rules we discussed in the chapter before and you will need to take regular insulin to cover protein amounts above 3oz/75g.

A final point – carbohydrate counting is not a precise science. Because we are recommending a diet of mainly natural foods, we do not know, for example, how big the apples you may choose to eat are – nor the size of the vegetables you have chopped up for use in recipes. The higher the carb intake you aim for, the more likely it is that you will make mistakes. Hopefully, though, those mistakes will be much smaller than the mistakes you might make attempting to calculate the carbs in the supposedly healthy, whole grain and low-fat standard recommended diet.

SAMPLE MENU PLAN – CARBOHYDRATE INTAKE LESS THAN 50G PER DAY

Day 1

BREAKFAST: 1 slice almond bread (in recipe section, Chapter 10), butter, 2 boiled eggs

10g carbs

LUNCH: Chicken in a cream and mushroom sauce, 5g carbs

Salad, 5g carbs

DINNER: Roast pork, 100g steamed new potatoes, 100g steamed broccoli, 25g carbs

100g mixed berries and 2tbsp double cream – 7g carbs

Daily totals: 47g carbs

Day 2:

BREAKFAST: Mushroom omelette made with two eggs and fried in butter, with two medium chopped tomatoes – 10g carbs

LUNCH: Baked salmon, mayonnaise and salad – 3g carbs

DINNER: Duck breast in Calvados (see recipe in Chapter 10), with 100g potatoes roasted in goose fat – 20g carbs

Cheddar cheese with one stick celery cut into strips, and 100g carrots cut into strips – 15g carbs

Daily totals: 48g carbs

Day 3:

BREAKFAST: Bacon and mushrooms (see recipe in chapter 8) – 3g carbs

LUNCH: Tuna Nicoise (see recipe in Chapter 10) – 5g carbs

DINNER: Roast beef with 1tbsp English mustard, 75g steamed carrots and 75g steamed green beans – 12g carbs

Cheese and 125g strawberries – 10g carbs

Daily totals: 30g carbs

Day 4:

BREAKFAST: Smoked salmon and scrambled eggs, with 1 medium finely chopped tomato 50g finely chopped red onions – 8g carbs

LUNCH: Home-made burgers with fried onions (see recipe in Chapter 10) and 80g bagged bistro salad, olive oil and white wine vinegar dressing – 10g carbs

DINNER: 2 medium chicken legs, roasted and home-made coleslaw (see recipe in Chapter 10) and 100g steamed green beans – 13g carbs

20g plain chocolate (70% cocoa solids) and 2tbsp hazelnuts – 15g carbs

Daily totals: 46g carbs

Day 5:

BREAKFAST: Asparagus Eggs – 4g carbs

LUNCH: Three slices ham and cauliflower cheese (see recipe in Chapter 10) – 15g carbs

DINNER: Lamb chops, 200g wilted spinach and butter, 100g carrots, cooked – 12g carbs

150g Strawberries and cheese – 12g carbs

Daily totals: 52g carbs

Day 6:

BREAKFAST: Low carb peanut/choc chip cookies x 3 (see recipe in Chapter 10) – 15g carbs

LUNCH: Prawn curry with 100g steamed broccoli (see recipe in Chapter 10) – 15g carbs

DINNER: Steak with your sauce of choice (see recipe in Chapter 10), cauliflower puree and salad – 10g carbs

Cheese and celery sticks (one stalk) – 3g carbs

Daily totals: 43 carbs

Day 7:

BREAKFAST: Smoked haddock, 2 poached eggs and 100g creamed spinach – 5g carbs

LUNCH: Cock- a- leekie soup (see recipe in Chapter 8), including rice – 10g carbs

DINNER: Scallops and black pudding with 100g steamed green beans – 10g carbs

Brie and a few grapes (6-7) – 5g carbs

Daily total: 30g carbs

If you want to follow a slightly higher carbohydrate diet, then the next sample menu is for you. Remember, if you want to increase your intake up to 130g add in carefully measured carbohydrates to meals in the form of potatoes, sweet potatoes, weighed portions of pasta or rice, or legumes.

SAMPLE MENU PLAN – CARBOHYDRATE INTAKE 50-90G A DAY

Day 1:

BREAKFAST: Omelette made with eggs, red pepper strips and cheese, with 125g potatoes chunks fried in olive oil – 25g carbs

LUNCH: Tuna Nicoise salad (see recipe in Chapter 10) and one medium slice of wholemeal bread and butter – 20g carbs

DINNER: Steak with your choice of sauce (see recipe in Chapter 10), salad and cauliflower puree

Cheese and an apple – 35g carbs

Daily total – 80g carbs

Day 2:

BREAKFAST: Greek yoghurt and berries (see recipe in Chapter 10) and a slice of almond bread – 25g carbs

LUNCH: Beef-burger with a slice of cheese and salad; an apple – 20g carbs

DINNER: Piri- Piri Chicken (see recipe in Chapter 10) with steamed green beans and a small baked potato (about 150g) – 35g carbs

Daily total – 80g carbs

Day 3:

BREAKFAST: Boiled eggs with asparagus and an orange – 17g carbs

LUNCH: Cajun salmon with lime mayonnaise, 150g steamed new potatoes and 100g steamed green beans – 37g carbs

DINNER: Italian lamb stew with rosemary and olives, 2 thin slices of garlic bread – 27g carbs

Daily total – 81g carbs

Day 4:

BREAKFAST: Bacon and eggs, potato scone and 100g mushrooms fried in butter – 20g carbs

LUNCH: Prawn curry with 100g steamed broccoli, 1 apple – 33g carbs

DINNER: Lamb steaks with yoghurt sauce (see recipe in Chapter 10) and sweet potato chips (100g) – 30g carbs

Daily total – 83g carbs

Day 5:

BREAKFAST: Scrambled eggs with 1 chopped tomato served on a slice of medium wholemeal bread – 18g carbs

LUNCH: Sliced ham, grated cheese and salad; 1 apple – 20g carbs

DINNER: Chicken in vermouth, cream and tarragon sauce, 100g peas, 1 slice low-carb Victoria sponge (see recipes for the chicken and the Victoria sponge in Chapter 10) – 30g carbs

Daily total – 68g carbs

Day 6:

BREAKFAST: Bacon and mushrooms (see recipe in Chapter 10) and an orange – 20g carbs

LUNCH: Roast chicken with pesto-griddled vegetables and 150g steamed new potatoes – 35g carbs

DINNER: Scallops and black pudding, 150g steamed broccoli, 1 apple and cheese – 25g carbs

Daily total – 80g carbs

Day 7:

BREAKFAST: Left over roast chicken and a piece of wholemeal toast – 15g carbs

LUNCH: Smoked salmon with a little cream cheese, and a cucumber salad, 1 apple – 20g carbs

DINNER: Prawn curry and 40g brown rice – 40g carbs

Daily total – 70g carbs

WHAT SHOULD I DRINK?

Water?

Okay, we all know the advice about drinking plenty of water and how good it is for you, but it can be difficult to do.

Obviously, if you are a coffee or tea drinker, then it depends on what you put in your tea or coffee. If you have it black and without sugar, then it is fine. If you drink it with milk, you ought to measure out how much milk you are putting in your tea and coffee, as milk does have carbohydrates in it (about 5g for 100ml). It is unlikely that you will be using very much milk, but you can keep the carb count as low as possible by using full cream milk or double cream. If you take sugar in your tea or coffee, then you need to swap this for a sweetener if you can't sacrifice the sweet taste.

Herbal teas are another alternative, and they have the added bonus of being caffeine-free.

While small quantities of milk are fine for tea and coffee, a glass of milk does have carbohydrates, and they will need to be taken into account to see if they fit into your planned carbohydrate intake for the day. We do not recommend fruit juices because the sugars from fruit juices go into your blood stream quickly and they are high carbohydrate drinks. The same applies to smoothies.

There are lots of sugar-free fizzy drinks out there. They will not have an adverse effect on your blood sugar, but the long-term effects on health of a regular intake of sweeteners are not known. Also, sugar-free fizzy drinks often contain lots of chemicals and artificial ingredients. One often raised complaint about artificial sweeteners is that they do nothing to re-educate your palate. They are very, very sweet and we are trying to steer ourselves away from a sweet tooth!

It is a good idea to carry Diastix or similar urine testing strips in your diabetes kit. In the old days, these were used to test urine, but now they are convenient to test "diet" drinks that are served draught rather than in a bottle or can. It is easy for bar staff to make errors in pouring drinks and you don't want an unexpected high blood sugar. You can reuse the same test strip in a session provided it does not change from blue (no sugar) to brown (sugar).

Energy drinks are often full of sugar, so do not drink them unless you are experiencing a hypo.

As for alcohol, aside from the usual health warnings, diabetics do need to exercise caution when drinking alcohol. You can read more about this in Chapter 9, but choose lower-sugar alcoholic beverages such as dry white and red wines, clear spirits such as gin or vodka served with a sugar-free mixer and steer clear of sugary cocktails, sweet and fortified wines, and beers and lagers.

CHAPTER 10

DELICIOUS LOW CARB RECIPES

This might be the best bit of the book for you as we're now going to talk about food, glorious food...

Sometimes, you need to engage a little bit of a different mindset when it comes to diabetes and the meals that you are going to be eating. We have been conditioned for many years to think that certain meals go along with certain times of the day – so cereal, for example, belongs to breakfast, sandwiches and soups are for lunch and meat, and two veg is your dinner option.

Puddings, of course, are often used by many people as a treat.

Broaden your horizons! Cereals, for example, are made by food manufacturers who have vast sums of money at their disposal to persuade you that pouring yourself a bowl of sugar-packed crap is somehow convenient and healthy. If you have ever taken a small child to the cinema, you will see that massive marketing machine in operation as children are bombarded with adverts for breakfast cereals which are inevitably sugar-covered.

So, resist those companies with their enormous advertising budgets trying to tell you that it is "natural" to eat cereal for breakfast. So, soup for breakfast? Hell, yeah. Leftover lamb stew which only needs a few moments heating up – that's convenient, isn't it?

Abandon your sandwiches for lunch theory too. Many commercially-available sandwiches can contain upwards of 45-50g of carbohydrate a pack, which eats into a huge chunk of your daily allowance without providing adequate amounts of protein or nutrients. Instead, opt for meat and salad, stews, fish dishes, soufflés or omelettes.

The picture we are trying to paint here is that breakfast, lunches and dinners do not need to be as strictly defined as convention dictates. Swap the three. If you are someone who does not have much of an appetite first thing and the thought therefore of stew for breakfast makes you faintly queasy, consider trying something light like a soft-boiled egg with cooked asparagus tips instead of the usual soldiers made from bread.

We do realise, however, that some ideas are too much of a break from the norm for everyone, so we've added in some adaptations of popular breakfast foods – such as pancakes, muffins and bread for you to try. We've also included low-carbohydrate baking for those of you in need of the occasional sweet treat.

Please note – carb counting isn't an exact science. It depends on self-measurement, the size of fruit and veg, the time of year because of the ripeness of produce and other factors, so carb counts for individual recipes cannot be exact. But because they are low in general, they give you a good idea of values.

Remember too, to take the protein into account if you are taking insulin. You will need 2 units of REGULAR insulin for every 3oz/75g (total weight of item) of lean protein.

Here are some general notes:

It is easier to double up quantities for recipes if you are serving for four instead of two than it is to divide recipes which is why we have suggested small serving sizes.

Most of the recipes take very little time to prepare and cook and are best made fresh. However, many of the main courses can be made in advance as this might make life easier for you.

You can change vegetable recommendations or suggestions for the cheese to your own preferences. In general, aubergines, green beans, courgettes, spring onions, mushrooms, spinach, kale and peppers are all low-carbohydrate vegetables for cooking with.

If you can find it and afford it, we recommend buying good quality meat from your butcher, fish from a fishmonger, eggs and cheese from a Farmer's Market, and organic fruit and veg. But such food can be much more expensive. If you can only buy one or two high-quality things, see our Appendix for what are the best choices to make if you are going to buy organic.

Remember, we have only provided a small selection of recipes here. There are many, many great low-carbohydrate cook books out there and a lot of recipes online. The recipes used on many of the American Paleo websites are also suitable for low-carbohydrate dieting so you might want to try these out as well. There is a full listing of further reading at the end of this book.

To minimise eye watering from cutting up onions, use a very sharp knife, on a chopping board and cut them as quickly as you can. Alternatively get your spouse to cut them! Chewing some strongly flavoured mint gum at the same time can also help.

To prevent your hands smelling of garlic or onions after cutting them, run your hands in cold water without rubbing them together. This prevents the odours cooking onto your hands. Then wash your hands normally with warm water and soap.

Ground almonds are perfect for baking. Unfortunately, they can also clog up your dishwasher so you are best to wash in a basin when you use them.

INTERESTING FACT

One study has shown that people who eat salad vegetables frequently, all year round, have a lower incidence of impaired glucose tolerance (13%) than those who eat them less often (17%).

Most impressive though was the incidence of type 2 diabetes, which was only 1% of those people eating salad vegetables regularly throughout the year compared with almost 6% of those individuals who ate them infrequently throughout the year.

The results for salad vegetable consumption remained significant after various adjustments even in people who were not overweight. Frequent fruit consumption was not significantly associated with lower diabetes incidence.

BREAKFAST RECIPES

Asparagus Eggs

Make this during peak asparagus season (roughly May to mid-June) with British asparagus, if at all possible, as that way you will get the most flavoursome asparagus.

1. 4 large, free-range eggs
2. 150g asparagus tips
3. Two rashers crispy bacon
4. 1 tbsp butter
5. Salt and freshly-ground black pepper

Place the four eggs in a small saucepan. Using boiling water from the kettle, pour over the four eggs to cover completely, place a lid on top and cook on top of the for four to five minutes. The water should come to the boil, turn it down and leave to simmer. Once the cooking time is completed, take the pan off the heat and run cold water over the eggs for two minutes.

Meanwhile, heat a griddle pan until very hot and melt the butter. Add the asparagus and the bacon and griddle until the veg is softened and the bacon very crispy. This should take about four minutes. Crumble the bacon rashers into small pieces.

Peel the eggs and place in egg cups. Slice the top of each and sprinkle the eggs with the bacon pieces, as well as a little seasoning. Serve two eggs per person along with the cooked asparagus to use as dippers for the eggs. Serves 2. CHO count per portion: 3g

Greek Yoghurt with Berries

Greek yoghurt contains more protein than ordinary yoghurt, making it more satisfying. This is a straightforward and quick breakfast for people who are time-pushed in the morning.

1. 400g full-fat Greek Yoghurt

2. 200g fresh berries – either blackberries, blueberries, raspberries or strawberries

3. 50g flaked almonds

Divide the yoghurt into two bowls and swirl in 100g of berries into each portion. Top each bowl with the flaked almonds. Serves 2. CHO per portion – 21g

Bacon and Eggs

This would not be a proper low-carbohydrate book without a mention of bacon and eggs! No doubt, many people will feel they do not really need a "recipe" for bacon and eggs, but try out this version anyway...

Buy the best quality bacon you can from outdoor roaming animals. Animals that live closer to the way nature intended produce the tastiest and healthiest meat, as well as living a life that is not cruel.

1. 4-6 rashers of back bacon

2. 4 eggs

3. 2tbsp double cream

4. 1tbsp butter

5. Salt and freshly-ground black pepper

6. 2 large tomatoes, halved

Crack the eggs into a bowl and stir well. Add salt and freshly-ground black pepper. Heat a large griddle pan on the hob. As bacon usually has enough fat, you should not need to add extra to the griddle pan. Cook the bacon – it will take roughly one minute or so each side, depending on how crispy you usually like it.

Add the tomato halves to the pan.

Meanwhile, in a small saucepan, add the butter and melt over a low heat, swirling to coat the pan. Add the eggs and move around the pan with a whisk, breaking up big lumps as you go. The eggs are cooked when all of the water has evaporated, but they will keep cooking when you take them off the heat so be careful not to let them get too dry. Mix in the cream, which will give a more luxurious feel to the dish.

Serve the bacon with the eggs and two tomato halves per person. Serves 2. CHO per portion: 6g

Dr. Katharine Morrison and Emma Baird

Bacon and Mushrooms

Mushrooms soak up bacon flavour really well. They make for a lovely combination.

1. 8 rashers of back bacon (or streaky, if that is your preference)
2. 200g mushrooms, sliced (use a mix of chestnut, button and Portobello for maximum flavour)
3. 4-5 stalks fresh thyme leaves only
4. 2tbsp butter

Melt the butter in a large frying pan. Add the mushrooms first and cook until softened and most of the water is evaporated. Add the thyme leaves and then add in the bacon which will take a minute or so on each side. Serves 2. CHO per portion: 5g

Low Carb Granola

1. 1 cup flax seeds

2. 1 cup sunflower seeds

3. 1 cup unsweetened shredded coconut

4. 1 cup chopped pecans

5. 1 cup chopped walnuts

6. 1 cup chopped almonds

7. 125g of butter melted

8. 2 teaspoons cinnamon

9. 2 teaspoons vanilla extract

Chop nuts in a food processor to the size you like. In a large roasting pan, mix together flax seeds, sunflower seeds, coconut and nuts. Drizzle with melted butter.

Stir in cinnamon, vanilla power and sugar substitute. Toast in the oven at 325 degrees for a half hour, stirring every 5 or 10 minutes.

For breakfast, add thick Greek yoghurt mixed with a little flax oil and double cream, and top with a few berries and toasted flaked almonds. Total CHO – 45g (amount will depend on portion size).

PUDDING IDEAS FOR GRANOLA

Granola is good mixed with melted butter as a chilled cheesecake base. To do this, chop to a very fine consistency.

It also makes a good crumble topping.

Mix some with extra ground almonds – about half and half, maybe some extra coconut too. Use raspberries as the base or stewed rhubarb or stewed apples and bake about 15 mins. This is good with low-carb custard, low-carb vanilla ice cream or lots of double cream.

Almond Bread

For two loaves:

1. 6 American cups ground almonds or 600g
2. 125g unsalted butter at room temperature (or melt in the microwave)
3. 500g mascarpone cheese
4. One teaspoon almond essence (can be left out)
5. 2 teaspoons baking powder
6. 1/2 teaspoon salt
7. 6 eggs

Preheat oven to 350 degrees F, or 180 C

In a mixer, cream the butter and mascarpone. Add the almond essence if using.

In a large bowl, mix ground almonds, baking soda and powder and salt.

Add the eggs to the wet ingredients then add the ground almonds a large spoonful at a time with the mixer going.

Grease a loaf pan (about 4 x 8 inches) generously with butter (or spray with non-stick cooking oil). Spoon batter into the pan, smoothing top. Bake at 350 F or 180C for 50-60 min (see note below) until lightly browned on top.

Remove from oven and allow to cool. Run a spatula around the sides of the pan, pressing gently against the loaf to loosen at the corners and bottom of the pan.

Wrap in tin foil. You can freeze these for weeks. Take out the night before you intend to use it. This is particularly good toasted. You can use with butter or sugar reduced jam/fruit spread. (Regular jam is 15g for a dessert spoon which is a typical serving size).

Each loaf yields 6 thick slices. CHO per slice – 6g

Muffins

Two muffins with fresh fruit and a good dollop of double cream make for a delicious and satisfying breakfast.

Preheat the oven to 160 degrees C for a fan oven and 180 degrees C for a standard oven. You will need a big bowl or jug and a smaller bowl or jug and one tablespoon, one fork, one teaspoon and one teacup, a muffin tin and 12 muffin cases.

Basic Mix:

Dry ingredients:

1. 1 cup soy flour
2. 1 cup ground almonds
3. 1 cup Splenda or granular sugar substitute
4. 2 heaped tablespoons of whey protein powder (optional)
5. Half a teaspoon of salt
6. 1 rounded teaspoon of baking powder
7. 1 rounded teaspoon of baking soda

Wet ingredients:

1. 1 cup of light cooking oil (light olive oil works well)
2. 2 large eggs
3. 1 cup double cream (can be soured or double or a mixture of both and can be tinned)
4. 2 tablespoons of water
5. 1 teaspoon vanilla essence

Mix the dry and wet ingredients separately and then add the dry to the wet.

Mixing with a spoon is fine. Add any extra ingredients you wish. A tablespoon of this mixture can be put into muffin cases to make 12 muffins.

Put in the warm oven for 12 minutes if a fan oven and 15 minutes in a standard oven. Check the muffins are cooked before switching off the oven by sticking a cocktail stick through the middle of one of them. If it comes out clean your muffins are ready. If not, put them in for a few more minutes and test again. These keep well in the fridge for a few days.

For variety:

1. Orange Muffins – add grated zest of two oranges.

2. Cherry Muffins – add chopped glace cherries.

3. Choc chip – add white, milk or plain chips.

4. Chocolate muffins – add 4 heaped teaspoons of cocoa powder to the dry ingredients.

5. Carrot – add a grated medium carrot and 2 rounded teaspoons of cinnamon powder.

CHO per muffin 10g (approximately it depends on what you add).

Scotch Pancakes

1. 2 large eggs separated
2. 60mls double cream
3. 1 teaspoon Splenda (or another granular sugar substitute)
4. Pinch of salt
5. 120 mg of ground almonds
6. ½ teaspoon of baking powder
7. Unsalted butter for frying

Put your frying pan or griddle on a low heat while you make the batter. (A thoroughly heated pan is the secret to good pancakes, and it avoids the bad first pancake scenario which we have all experienced.)

Beat the egg whites till stiff. An electric whisk is best.

In another bowl mix the egg yolks, cream, sweetener, salt and baking powder.

Add the ground almonds and beat until smooth.

Add some of the egg whites to the almond mixture and mix. Fold in the rest of the egg whites in batches. A large metal spoon is best.

Now raise the temperature under the frying pan. Put some butter in the pan and when it sizzles, add a large spoonful of the batter. For a 24-inch frying pan, you can make three pancakes at once.

Put the spoonful of batter in the pan. Don't touch the pancake until bubbles have formed on the top of the pancake and it has risen a little. This will take about three minutes. When bubbles have formed on the top turn and cook for about another two minutes. Add more butter as needed between batches.

These keep well in the fridge for a few days. CHO per pancake – 3g

EGG RECIPES

Courgette and Pepper Frittata

A frittata is basically a substantial omelette, which is perfect for lunch or dinner. Or breakfast too, if you wake up hungry. You can swap in different vegetables to suit your own preferences, and we have added in some suggestions below.

1. 6 large, fresh free-range eggs

2. 2tbsp butter or olive oil

3. 1 medium-sized courgette, sliced into even-sized discs

4. 1 red pepper, cut into strips

5. 2 spring onions, sliced

6. 50g freshly grated Parmesan or cheddar cheese, grated

7. Salt and freshly-ground black pepper

Preheat the oven to 180 degrees C. Melt the butter (or heat the olive oil) in a large, oven-proof frying pan/omelette pan and add the vegetables to the pan. Cook until softened – about five minutes. Whisk the eggs together and add to the pan, tilting to coat. Allow the bottom to cook for a few minutes and then sprinkle the top with the grated cheese. Bake in the oven for 10 minutes, until the top has set.

This is great served with a green salad or steamed green beans. Serves 2. CHO per portion – 9g.

Other suggestions:

1. 100g sliced mushrooms, instead of the courgette

2. 50g chopped ham, instead of or with the cheese

3. 100g chopped fine beans, instead of the courgette

4. 75g pancetta, chopped with the Parmesan

Baked Eggs

Eggs are a crucial part of a low-carbohydrate diet -and with good reason. An egg is a very nutritious food, packed with protein, vitamins A, D and B2, as well as iodine. There are lots of diverse ways to eat eggs, so even if you don't like them one way – the boiled egg, for example – then soufflés, omelettes or recipes which use eggs as a thickener might be for you.

1. 4 large, free-range eggs
2. 4 rashers back bacon
3. 2tbsp double cream
4. Salt and freshly-ground black pepper
5. Butter

Preheat the oven to 180 degrees C. Rub four ramekin dishes with a little butter and press the bacon rashers into the ramekins so that they form a circle in the dish. Break each egg into the ramekin (the yolk should hopefully remain intact) and add a little seasoning to each plate. The dishes should not need much seasoning because the bacon is salty. Add a half tbsp of double cream to each ramekin and bake in the oven for 10 minutes.

NOTE – you can also use a muffin tin to bake the eggs if you do not have ramekin dishes. CHO per portion – negligible.

Devilled Eggs

These are surprisingly addictive!

1. Six eggs

2. Mayonnaise – a couple of squirts

3. Salt

4. Pepper

5. A small quantity of either horseradish sauce or Tabasco or chilli flakes.

Boil the eggs till they are hard boiled. This means six minutes or more at a rolling boil.

Let them cool. Take the shells off and cut in half-length ways. Take out the yolks. Mash the yolks up with any of your hot ingredients plus the seasoning and mayonnaise. You want enough mayonnaise to get to a soft but not sloppy consistency. Put the yolk mixture back into the holes in the egg whites.

Cover with cling film and put in the fridge for 30 minutes or more. Enjoy. (These also make excellent canapés.) CHO count per serving – negligible.

MAIN COURSES

FISH/SEAFOOD

Prawn Curry

1. 1tbsp coconut oil

2. 50g creamed coconut, chopped into small pieces*

3. 200g king prawns

4. 5-6 spring onions, sliced

5. 1 clove garlic, crushed

6. 2tbsp fresh-grated ginger

7. 1tbsp turmeric

8. 1-2 fresh chillies (keep the seeds in if you like hot curries)

9. 1 tin chopped tomatoes

Melt the coconut oil in a large wok. Add the spring onions and cook for 2-3 minutes. Add the garlic, ginger and chillies and stir fry for another minute or so. Add the tinned tomatoes and the chopped creamed coconut. Fill the empty tomato tin with cold water and add to the pan, along with the turmeric. Bring the mixture to the boil and simmer for ten to 15 minutes (the longer you simmer, the thicker and the more concentrated your sauce will be). Add the prawns and warm through – about one to two minutes. It is very easy to overcook prawns so do not allow the mixture to boil fiercely after adding the prawns. Serves 2. CHO per portion – 12g

NOTE – Barts Spices creamed coconut sachets contain the least carbohydrate per portion.

Tuna Nicoise

Traditionally, Tuna Nicoise is made with potatoes, but we're going to miss them out for this salad. We've suggested tinned tuna for convenience/price, but do add in fresh tuna if you prefer – one steak per person, and fry it on a griddle for approximately two minutes on each side.

1. 2 x tins tuna canned in spring water
2. 100g fine green beans
3. 50g pitted black olives
4. 2 eggs
5. 2 little gem lettuces
6. 3tbsp extra virgin olive oil
7. 1tbsp fresh lemon juice
8. 1tbsp whole grain mustard
9. Salt and freshly-ground black pepper

Put the eggs in a saucepan and add boiling water. Bring back to a simmer, cover the pan and cook for five to seven minutes (a soft-boiled egg makes for a nicer contrast of textures, but if you prefer firmer yolks, boil for a longer time).

Slice the green beans in half and for the last three minutes of the eggs' cooking time, add them to the egg pan.

Whisk together the oil, lemon juice, mustard and salt and pepper. Chop the little gem lettuces and divide between two plates. Drain the tinned tuna and flake over the lettuce, along with the olives.

Once the eggs and green beans are finished, remove the eggs from the pan and place under running water for two minutes. Peel the shells, slice the eggs in two and add the halves to the plate. Drain the beans and place on a plate. Drizzle over the dressing and serve. Serves 2. CHO per portion – 5g

Scallops with Black Pudding or Chorizo

This is a lovely luxury dish. Black pudding contains more carbohydrate than chorizo because it is made with oats, but we are only using it here in small quantities. If you are going to use black pudding, we recommend Stornoway black pudding, which can be bought online as well as from good butchers.

1. 8 medium-sized scallops

2. 6 spring onions, sliced finely

3. Salt and freshly-grounded black pepper

4. 100g black pudding, sliced

5. 2tbsp butter

Melt 1tbsp of the butter in a saucepan and add the spring onions. Cook until softened and then remove from the pan with a slotted spoon. Add the other tbsp of butter and cook the scallops for one minute on each side. Remove from the pan and keep warm. Remove the plastic coating from the black pudding and add to the pan along with the spring onions. It will disintegrate but move around the pan for a few minutes until cooked through.

Plate up four scallops on two plates and scatter the black pudding and spring onions on the top.

This is good served with steamed spinach or broccoli.

NOTE – to make this using chorizo, buy cooking chorizo and chop into small dice. Cook until the red oils run from the sausage pieces and they are lightly browned. Mix with the spring onions and scatter over the scallops as before. Serves 2. CHO per portion – 10g

Cajun Salmon with Lime Mayonnaise

1. 2tsp Cajun seasoning
2. 3tbsp mayonnaise
3. 1 lime
4. 4 salmon fillets
5. 1 garlic clove crushed
6. 1tbsp extra virgin olive oil

Heat the oven to 180C/160C fan/gas 4. Place the seasoning on a plate and use to dust the salmon fillets, shaking off any excess. Heat an oven-proof frying pan.

Add half the oil and sear the salmon, skin-side down, for 30 secs, then turn over and cook for 1 min. Transfer to the oven and roast for 6 mins until tender, but still very moist in the middle.

Put the mayonnaise in a bowl and beat in the remaining oil with the garlic. Add a light grating of lime zest, then cut the lime in half and add a squeeze of the juice. Serves 4. CHO per person 4g

WHITE MEAT

Roast Chicken with Pesto-griddled Vegetables

Remember, don't throw away the chicken carcass as it can be used to make the most delicious (and nutritious) chicken stock. If you can't eat roast meat without gravy, there is also a suggestion for a low-carbohydrate gravy in the sauces/miscellaneous section.

1. 1.5kg chicken (free-range and preferably organic)
2. Salt and freshly-ground black pepper
3. 6tbsp butter
4. 1 lemon
5. 1tbsp fresh sage leaves, chopped
6. 4 cloves garlic
7. 2 courgettes
8. 1 aubergine
9. 1 red pepper
10. 1 red onion
11. 1tbsp olive oil
12. 6tbsp fresh pesto sauce (for our home-made recipe see further on).

Preheat the oven to 200 degrees C. Take your chicken out of the fridge and remove all of the packaging. Mix the butter with the sage, salt and butter and rub all over the chicken. Half the lemon and place it in the chicken body cavity.

Place the chicken in a roasting dish and cover with foil. Roast in the oven for an hour and a half (or whatever the instructions say on your bird), removing the foil for the last 15 minutes so the skin browns and crisps up nicely.

Take the chicken from the oven and cover with foil. Leave to rest for 20 minutes, while you get on with the griddled veg. Cut the vegetables into evenly-sized portions and heat a griddle pan or frying pan. Add the olive oil and cook the vegetables in batches (if you put too many in the pan at once they will stew instead of frying). Put aside the cooked vegetables as they cook into a large bowl. When all the vegetables are cooked, add the fresh pesto and mix well to cook. Serve the chicken with a portion of the pesto vegetables. Serves 4-6. CHO per portion for 4 – 7g. CHO per portion for 6 – 5g

Chicken in a Vermouth, Cream and Tarragon Sauce.

1. Chicken pieces skinned, preferably on the bone, e.g. thighs.

2. 75g Butter

3. A wine glass of dry white vermouth

4. 2tbsp Tarragon or cider vinegar

5. Leaves from a small bunch of tarragon or use dried

6. 300mls double cream

7. A squeeze of lemon juice

You may add leeks or mushrooms to the sauce as well if you like.

Season the chicken with salt and pepper. Melt the butter in a large frying pan or wok and lightly brown the chicken in the wok. Remove the chicken. If you are using leeks or mushrooms, fry them now and then remove.

Discard most of the remaining butter and put the wok back on the heat. Add the vermouth and vinegar and scrape down the pan. Reduce the vermouth for a few minutes then add the cream. Stir and then add the chicken and vegetables back in.

Gently simmer for 20 minutes with the lid partially on to allow further reduction of the sauce. Add more vermouth if it is getting too thick.

Just before serving, add a light squeeze of lemon. Serve with green vegetables to mop up the sauce. Serves 4. CHO per portion – 4g

Piri Piri Chicken

1. 2 red chillies, halved, seeded and finely chopped
2. 1 red pepper, halved, seeded and roughly chopped
3. 3tbsp red wine vinegar
4. 4 tbsp olive oil
5. 4 boneless chicken breasts

Tip the chillies and pepper into a food processor, add vinegar, oil and seasoning. Whizz until chunky.

Slash the chicken breasts across skin side and put in a shallow oven proof dish. Pour over three-quarters of pepper marinade, turn chicken to coat it. Reserve the remaining marinade.

Marinate for at least 10 mins, or overnight if you have the time.

Heat a griddle or heavy frying pan, add chicken and cook for 5-6 mins on each side, turning once. Serve on a bed of salad leaves with the reserved marinade drizzled over. Serves 4. CHO per portion – 3g

Easy Chicken Caesar Salad *(courtesy of Fergus Craig)*

This summer staple takes very little time to put together so you can soak up the summer evening sun instead.

To make it the easy way, use Cardini's Caesar dressing from the very man who invented the thing and an amazingly low 1.4g carbohydrate per 100g. The walnuts are the perfect replacement for the usual croutons, giving the dish a lovely contrast of texture. If you prefer pecans that would also work, though they are a bit higher in carbs than walnuts (13g per 100g as opposed to 3g).

Oh, and the Parmesan shavings also give the opportunity to use that potato peeler which you might have thought had gone into early retirement when you took up the low-carb diet...

1. 1 Romaine lettuce (or Cos)

2. 1/3 bottle Cardini's Caesar dressing

3. 3 anchovies, sliced finely

4. 1 roast chicken breast, sliced

5. A handful of walnut pieces

6. Parmesan shavings

Shred the Romaine lettuce crossways and put half in a large bowl. Pour on half the dressing and mix well.

Now add the rest of the lettuce, anchovies and walnuts and mix again. Pour over the remaining dressing and arrange the chicken slices on top.

Finally, scatter the Parmesan shavings over the top and enjoy. Serves 1. CHO per portion – 2-3g

Homemade Hamburgers

Burgers can vary widely in carbohydrate content, depending on how much filler in the form of breadcrumbs the manufacturer puts in. The higher quality burgers available from butchers and supermarkets can contain less of these fillers, but to be really sure – why not make your own burgers?

We suggested a filler of ground almonds (although you can leave this out), which adds vitamin E and fibre to the dish.

Obviously, these are burgers without the bun or chips, but a well-made burger with a great topping tastes great on its own.

1. 500g steak mince

2. 300g pork mince

3. 1 small onion, finely chopped

4. 2tbsp olive oil

5. 2 cloves garlic, crushed

6. 50g ground almonds

7. 2 medium eggs, free-range

8. 4-6 sprigs thyme (leaves only)

9. 1 stalk rosemary, leaves only

10. Salt and freshly-ground black pepper

Fry the onion in 1tbsp of the olive oil – it should only take a few minutes. Add the garlic at the end and cook for another 30 seconds. Allow to cool. Finely chop the thyme and rosemary. Mix the onions with the meat, chopped herbs, ground almonds and beaten eggs. The easiest way to do this is to use your hands as that allows you to distribute everything throughout the meat mixture. Shape into eight burgers. (If you make home-made burgers a lot, it is worth buying a burger press.) Chill in the fridge for half an hour.

Fry or griddle the burgers (three or four minutes each side – no pink juices should run out when you press down on the burgers) and serve with some of the suggestions below as toppings.

Fried onions for four burgers

1. 1 large onion, sliced

2. 2bsp butter

Melt the butter and fry the onions slowly and gently until lightly-browned (about 15 minutes) Season with salt and use to top the burgers.

Cheese burgers – top each burger with sliced cheese. Gherkins will also help cut through the richness of the burgers.

For spicy burgers, add a chopped chilli to the meat mixture and top each burger with 1-2tbsp home-made guacamole. (Recipe further on). Makes 8 burgers. CHO per burger – 3g. Fried onion topping 1g. Cheese and gherkin topping 2g. Home-made guacamole topping 3g

RED MEAT

Meatloaf

1. 1kg steak mince (from the butcher for better quality)
2. 1 large onion, very finely chopped
3. 2-3 stalks of celery, very finely chopped
4. 2 cloves garlic, crushed
5. 2 small chillies, finely chopped
6. 60g ground almonds
7. 2 large eggs
8. 40g Parmesan cheese, grated
9. 4-6 rashers streaky bacon
10. Salt and pepper

Preheat the oven to 180 degrees C. Mix all the ingredients (except the bacon) in a large bowl. The easiest way to do this is with your hands, scrunching everything together until it is well combined. Grease a 2lb loaf tin and pack the mix in (you may also need another dish). Top with the rashers of bacon. Cover with foil and bake in the oven for 60 minutes. Take the foil off for the last five minutes of cooking time to brown the top.

There will be plenty of juices so serve slices of the meatloaf with spoonfuls of the juices. It goes well with steamed green vegetables – either broccoli, spinach or green beans. Serves 6. CHO per portion – 5g

Lamb Steaks with Yoghurt Sauce

Lamb can be overlooked by many people, who find the meat fatty. It is, however, delicious, with a sweet flavour that can be much more interesting than beef. This Greek-inspired dish could be served with the aubergine and courgette stacks (recipe further on) or a salad with tahini dressing (recipe further on) to continue the Greek theme.

1. 4 lamb leg steaks

2. Olive oil

3. 3-4 sprigs thyme, leaves only

4. Salt and freshly-ground black pepper

5. 250g full-fat Greek yoghurt

6. 80g cucumber

7. 1 clove garlic, crushed

8. Few mint leaves, finely chopped

Take the lamb steaks out of the fridge half an hour before you want to cook them. Finely chop the thyme leaves and mix with the salt and pepper. Add to 1-2tbsp of the olive oil and rub into the lamb steaks. Set aside.

Scoop the seeds out of the cucumber, using a teaspoon and chop into small dice. Add the cucumber, garlic and mint to the yoghurt, along with a little salt and a generous amount of freshly-ground black pepper. Mix well.

Cook the lamb steaks on either a griddle or in a frying pan for four to five minutes each side (or according to the packet instructions). Top each steak with a generous spoonful of the yoghurt topping. Serves 4. CHO per portion – 4g

Italian Lamb Stew with Rosemary and Olives
1. 1.25kg lamb shoulder, trimmed of fat
2. olive oil
3. 2 celery stalks, diced
4. 2 cloves garlic, sliced
5. 1tbsp rosemary, chopped
6. 10 pitted black olives
7. small bunch chopped parsley, chopped
8. 1½ large onions, chopped
9. 2 carrots diced
10. 175mls white wine
11. 400g tinned tomatoes
12. 1 lemon zested and chopped

Heat the oven to 160C/140C fan/gas 3.

Cut the lamb into chunks. Heat 1tbsp oil in a large, oven-proof casserole dish. Brown the meat all over in batches (if you put too much meat in the pan when browning, you end up stewing the meat instead). Pour in 2tbsp of olive oil and add the onions, celery, carrots, garlic and rosemary.

Season and cook for 10 min. Add the wine, tomatoes and meat and bring to a simmer. Cover and cook in the oven for 2½ -3 hrs until tender. If you need to thicken the sauce, remove the veg & lamb and boil until you get the required consistency, then put veg & meat back into the dish.

Stir in the olives and lemon juice, sprinkle with the lemon zest and parsley and serve. Serves 4. CHO per portion – 17g

Moussaka

Ingredients

1. 1tbsp olive oil, plus extra for brushing
2. 1 large onion, finely chopped
3. 2 garlic cloves, crushed
4. 500g lamb mince
5. 2 tbsp tomato purée
6. ½ tsp ground cinnamon
7. 400g can chopped tomatoes
8. 2tsp dried oregano
9. 600g (about 2 medium) aubergines

For the topping:

1. 150ml Greek yoghurt
2. 1 medium egg, beaten
3. 25g freshly grated Parmesan
4. 50g feta

Heat the oil in a large frying pan over a medium heat. Add the onion and garlic and cook, stirring, for five minutes, until soft. Increase the heat, add the minced lamb and cook, stirring, for five minutes, until browned. Drain off the fat in a sieve, then return the meat to the pan.

Add the purée and cinnamon and cook, stirring, for one minute. Add the tomatoes, then half-fill the can with water and pour into the pan. Add the oregano, season, and bring to the boil. Reduce the heat and simmer, occasionally stirring, for 20 minutes.

Meanwhile, preheat the grill to medium-high. Cut each aubergine diagonally into 5mm-thick slices. Brush with oil, put half on a baking sheet and grill for five minutes, turning halfway, until pale golden. Drain on kitchen paper while grilling the remainder.

Preheat the oven to 200°C/fan180°C/gas 6. For the topping, mix the yoghurt, egg and half the cheeses. Season with pepper.

Spread half the lamb mixture in a deep, 1.2-litre oven-proof dish. Overlap with half the aubergine and the rest of the lamb. Top with rest of the aubergine, spoon over yoghurt mixture and scatter with the remaining cheeses. Bake for 35 minutes or until golden and bubbling. Serves 4. CHO per portion – 12g

Shepherd's Pie *(courtesy of Fergus Craig)*

This is a fantastic winter favourite and proof that comfort food doesn't have to be laden with starchy carbs. It's almost worth having winter if you can enjoy this with family and friends around the table.

1. 1 cauliflower, florets steamed till soft

2. 500g lamb mince

3. 1 red onion, finely chopped

4. 1 carrot, thinly sliced

5. 1 stick celery, sliced

6. 2 cloves garlic, crushed

7. A handful of grated gruyere cheese

8. 2tbsp tomato purée

9. A good slug of Worcestershire sauce

10. 1tbsp olive oil

11. Salt & freshly ground black pepper

In a large pan, heat the oil then add the onion, carrot and celery. Five minutes over a medium heat will soften them nicely. Add the garlic and cook for a further minute. Now add the lamb and cook until nicely browned. Add the tomato purée, Worcester sauce and seasoning to taste.

As the lamb is simmering, put the softened cauliflower and cheese into a food processor and whizz until you have a nice smooth consistency. Season to taste.

Place the lamb mixture in a deep baking dish and smooth the cauliflower over the top. Bake in the oven for around 30 minutes at 170 degrees (fan) until golden and bubbling. Serves 4. CHO per portion – 14g

Steaks with Different Sauces

Again, it would be difficult to write a low-carbohydrate diet book without including a steak recipe. It may be a cliché when it comes to low-carb eating, but that doesn't mean it's any less worthwhile including. Steak is an individual preference; whether that is the cut of meat or how long it is cooked for. You can use cheaper cuts – rump or sirloin, rather than fillet – and for maximum flavour, rib-eye as it is fattier. Purists would cook it rare, but many people do baulk at the sight of bloody meat, so cook it how you, and your guests, please.

Again, meat that comes from grass-fed animals and that has been left to hang for a long time is the healthiest and delicious choice, but it can be pretty expensive. Think of steak, therefore, as an occasional treat.

1. 2 x 150-200g steaks of your choice
2. Salt and freshly-ground black pepper
3. 1 tbsp olive oil
4. 1 tbsp butter

Take your steaks out of the fridge 30 minutes before you want to cook them to allow them to come to room temperature. Pat them dry with kitchen paper, as plastic packaging tends to make the meat wet. Rub them with the olive oil and season both sides generously with salt and pepper.

To cook them, heat either a griddle pan (you will get aesthetically-pleasing grill marks this way) or heavy-based frying pan as hot as you can and add the steaks. For rare steaks, cook them for roughly 2 minutes each side, for medium steaks, cook them for three minutes and for well-done steaks approximately four minutes. Add the butter for the last 30 seconds of cooking as this will add flavour.

Once the steaks are done to your liking, remove from the pan and cover with foil to keep warm. In the meantime, get on with your favoured sauce.

Mushroom and brandy sauce

1. 150g finely chopped mushrooms
2. 1 clove garlic, crushed
3. 2tbsp brandy
4. 150ml double cream

Add the finely chopped mushrooms to the pan and cook for three to four minutes. Add the garlic and cook for a further minute. Add the brandy, turn up the heat and cook until the brandy has evaporated. Add the cream and bring the sauce to the boil. Season to taste.

If a cream sauce is too rich for you, you can also serve your steak with fried mushrooms (150g for two people, fried in the pan juices with a little extra butter) or fried mushrooms, again fried in the pan juices and a little extra butter.

For a really fresh option, you can also serve steaks with salsa. Make this a few hours beforehand to give the flavours plenty of time to develop.

1. 4 large tomatoes
2. 1 clove garlic, crushed
3. 1 green chilli, de-seeded and sliced
4. 2tbsp fresh coriander, chopped
5. ½ small onion, finely diced
6. ½ lime, juiced
7. Salt and pepper

Peel and deseed the tomatoes – you can peel them by marking crosses in the tomatoes with a sharp knife, pouring boiling water over them and leaving them for a minute. The skins should then peel off easily. Then cut the tomatoes in half and squeeze over the sink to remove the seeds (or you can scoop them out with a teaspoon).

Finely chop the tomato halves and mix with the garlic, green chilli, coriander, onion, lime juice and seasoning.

If you choose this topping for your steak, it goes well with a little gem lettuce and avocado salad. Serves 2. CHO per serving – Mushroom and brandy sauce 3g. Fried onions – 3g. Fried mushrooms – 3g. Salsa – 7g

Lamb Mince Curry

Takeaway curries can include extra sugar, cheap vegetable oils, fillers such as potatoes and of course the obligatory rice and naan bread, all of which result in a dish which is high in carbohydrates.

Here, however, we have made a curry which is fresh and which makes the most of the health-giving properties of spices such as cinnamon, turmeric, coriander and black pepper[110].

1. 500g lamb mince
2. 2tbsp coconut oil or ghee
3. 1 onion, finely sliced
4. 2 cloves garlic, crushed
5. 2 fresh chillies, sliced (keep the seeds in if you prefer hot curries)
6. 2tbsp freshly-grated ginger
7. 1 stick cinnamon
8. 2tbsp coriander seeds
9. 2tbsp black peppercorns
10. 1tbsp ground cumin
11. 2tbsp turmeric
12. 1 tin chopped tomatoes
13. 100g frozen peas

In a small, heavy-based saucepan, dry-fry the coriander seeds and black peppercorns for a few minutes until you start to smell them. Set aside to cool and then pound with a pestle or mortar until ground. You can also use a coffee grinder to do this job (although you will never again be able to use it to grind coffee beans unless you want really peculiar-tasting coffee).

Heat the coconut oil or ghee in a large saucepan or wok and add the mince. Cook until browned, stirring regularly to break up any big clumps. This should take up to 10 minutes. Add the onions, garlic, ginger, chillies and cook for another two minutes.

Add the coriander, black pepper, cumin, turmeric and the cinnamon stick and cook for another two minutes. Add the tomatoes, bring to a simmer and allow to cook gently for half an hour. You may need to add extra water. Five minutes before the end of the cooking time, add the peas. Serves 4. CHO per serving – 13g

SOUPS

Broccoli and Stilton Soup

This is a classic soup – delicious, satisfying and suitable for winter.

1. 2tbsp butter
2. 1 small onion, peeled and diced
3. 2 cloves garlic, crushed
4. 1kg broccoli, chopped (stalk and all)
5. 175g Stilton cheese, crumbled
6. 1-litre fresh chicken stock
7. 1tsp dried Italian herbs
8. Salt and freshly-ground black pepper

Melt the butter in a large stockpot/saucepan. Add the onion and fry gently until translucent. Add the crushed garlic and the broccoli and mix well. Shake in the tsp of herbs and add the fresh chicken stock.

Bring to a simmer, cover the saucepan and cook for five minutes until the broccoli is soft. Add the crumbled Stilton and simmer for a few more minutes. Use a stick blender to blend the soup to a smooth purée and season to taste (you may not need much salt because Stilton is very salty). Serves 4. CHO per portion – 7g

Onion Soup

Most of the time, traditional onion soup is served with bread and cheese floating on top, which obviously puts the carbohydrate count up considerably. However, without the bread, this is still a delicious and nutritious soup, which can be served as a starter.

1. 1kg onions, peeled, halved and finely sliced

2. 4-5 sprigs thyme, leaves only

3. 1-litre fresh chicken stock (see recipe further on)

4. 1 glass (125ml) dry white wine

5. 2tbsp butter

6. Salt and freshly-ground black pepper

7. Shavings of fresh Parmesan cheese (optional)

Melt the butter in a large saucepan/stockpot and add the onions. Fry gently, with occasional stirring to prevent sticking for 15-20 minutes until the onions are softened and slightly caramelised. Add the thyme and the wine and bring to the boil.

Reduce the wine volume by half by continuing to boil and then add the stock. Bring to the boil again and then reduce the heat and allow the soup to simmer for five minutes or so.

Add seasoning to taste (home-made stock does not contain salt) and sprinkle each bowlful with shavings of Parmesan cheese. Serves 6. CHO per portion 5g

Cream of Mushroom Soup

1. 50g butter
2. 1 large onion
3. 4-6 large portabella mushrooms or equivalent
4. ½ pint double cream
5. ½ glass sherry
6. ½ pint chicken stock

Place the butter in a saucepan and melt. Add the chopped onion and fry till soft, then add the chopped mushrooms and fry.

Add the stock. Simmer till mushrooms and onions both very soft. Allow to cool. Take a hand-held blender and pulverise till your soup is a creamy consistency.

Leave till 10 minutes before you are ready to serve. Put the soup back on the heat, add the sherry and cream and warm it up while stirring gently. You can prepare the soup the day before if you like, store it in the fridge and finish off just before serving.

The same method works for almost all cream soups. Fry your onion in butter, add a vegetable, add stock, then pulverise, and then add cream just before serving.

Celery soup is done by this method, but the sherry is omitted. For cream of tomato soup, add tinned tomatoes in juice after the onions/ butter but use far less stock, if any. Add chopped basil just before serving.

For vegetable broths, where you are adding chicken, add pre-cooked chicken for a clear soup. You can add raw chicken and cook it in the soup, but it will make the liquor cloudy.

Slow cookers are particularly good for soups. Just put in your ingredients, making sure there is stock nearly up to the brim, switch on, and the next day or later that day your soup is ready. Many soups and stews taste better if they are made a day or so in advance of serving them. Serves 4. CHO per portion – 5g

VEGETABLE RECIPES

Tomato, Mozzarella and Basil Salad

This is a classic Italian salad, known as Insalata Caprese. It is best made from the freshest seasonal tomatoes you can buy – or even better, home-grown, either in your own garden or a great local nursery. The secret with tomatoes is to take them out of the fridge an hour or so before you want to eat them, as the cold kills tomato flavour.

1. 4 medium to large-sized tomatoes

2. 1pkt fresh Mozzarella (about 150-200g) cheese

3. 8-10 fresh basil leaves

4. Extra virgin olive oil (preferably of Italian origin)

5. Salt and freshly-ground black pepper

Slice the tomatoes evenly and divide among four side plates. Arrange with slices of the fresh Mozzarella (overlapping is pretty) and roughly rip the basil leaves, scattering these between the four dishes. Drizzle each plate with a little extra-virgin olive oil and season each plate with salt and freshly-ground black pepper. Serves 4. CHO per portion – 5g

Guacamole with Vegetable Crudités

This is our version of crisps 'n' dips – a smooth, flavoursome dip, served with fresh, crunchy vegetables so that you get the necessary contrast in textures. Avocados are jam-packed with healthy nutrients – potassium, fibre, and vitamins C, E and K.

1. 1 large, ripe avocado
2. 2tbsp good quality mayonnaise
3. 1 fresh chilli, seeds removed and sliced
4. 1 clove garlic, crushed
5. 1 medium tomato chopped
6. Half a lime, juice only
7. Salt and freshly-ground black pepper

Crudités:

1. 1-2 sticks celery, cut into batons
2. 1 red pepper, cut into strips
3. 1 green pepper, cut into strips

Scoop out the avocado and place in a large bowl with all of the other ingredients, except for the seasoning. You can either use a hand blender to blend this together (you'll get a smoother dip this way) or a potato masher/fork with give you a chunky textured dip. Season to taste with salt and pepper.

Place the dip in a bowl and serve with the fresh crudités for dipping. Serves 4. CHO per portion 7.5g

Courgette, Aubergine and Halloumi Stacks

1. 1 large courgette, sliced into even-sized discs

2. 1 large aubergine, sliced into even-sized discs

3. 1pkt Halloumi cheese

4. 1tsp chilli flakes

5. 1tsp dried Italian herbs

6. Salt and freshly-ground black pepper

7. Salad leaves to serve

8. 3tbsp olive oil

Preheat the oven to 180 degrees C. Lay the courgette and aubergine on a baking tray (you may need two so that the slices can all lie flat) and sprinkle with 2tbps of the olive oil, the Italian herbs and salt and pepper. Cook in the oven for 10-15 minutes until lightly browned.

Meanwhile, heat a griddle pan and cut the Halloumi cheese into thick slices. Brush the cheese with the last tbsp of oil and chilli flakes. Fry the cheese until golden.

Divide the salad leaves between four plates. Starting with an aubergine disc, layer the stacks on each plate aubergine/courgette/ Halloumi until everything has been used up. Serves 4, CHO per serving – 10g

Low-Carb Coleslaw

For portions of roast chicken or home-made burgers, coleslaw makes a lovely accompaniment. Many commercial versions can be high in carbohydrate because manufacturers add sugar to the dressings and use a lot of carrot – which is greater in carbohydrates than other veggies.

Also, commercial versions often use cheap and nasty vegetable oils for their mayonnaise, which we want to avoid because of their inflammatory behaviour on the body.

1. ½ white cabbage, sliced finely (about 300g)

2. ½ medium-sized carrot, peeled and thickly grated (about 100g)

3. 2-3 spring onions, chopped

4. ½ medium-sized courgette, cut into fine matchsticks (about 100g)

5. 8tbsp good-quality mayonnaise (see the home-made recipe for mayonnaise later on)

6. Salt and freshly-ground black pepper

Mix together the first five ingredients in a large bowl. Add the seasoning to taste. Leave for half an hour to allow the flavours to mingle properly. Makes 4-6 servings. CHO per portion – 8g if serving four, 5g if serving 6

NOTE – home-made coleslaw does not have the same lasting qualities as the commercial stuff because it doesn't contain the same nasty chemicals. You can, however, keep it for a day or two in the fridge. You will just need to stir well before serving again as it will start to separate.

Cauliflower Mash

1. Head of cauliflower cut into its florets
2. 1oz butter
3. Double cream
4. Salt and pepper

Optional (depending on preferences):

1. Fried onions or shallots
2. Cooked ham or pancetta in strips/cubes
3. Grated cheddar cheese mixed in or as a topping

Steam your cauliflower or cook in boiling water in a saucepan till it is very soft but has not yet started to disintegrate.

Put the drained cooked cauliflower into a bowl and add the butter. Add some double cream. Mash up with a potato masher. The consistency you want may vary. The more cream, the softer your finished dish will be. Add your other desired ingredients – onions, ham and cheese or herbs.

This cauliflower mash can be used in dishes where you would previously have used mashed potato, such as shepherd's pie or as an accompaniment to the main dish. Serves 4. CHO per portion – 5g

Buttered Peas and Leeks

1. 2 leeks, very finely sliced
2. 1tbsp olive oil
3. 250g frozen peas
4. 2 spring onions, sliced finely
5. 15g butter
6. 200mls vegetable stock

Gently soften the leeks in butter and oil in a pan for 15-20 minutes until almost meltingly soft. (This can be done a day ahead. Just reheat before continuing recipe.)

Stir in the stock, bring to a simmer and cook, occasionally stirring, for five minutes. Stir in the peas and onions for 3-5 minutes until the peas are defrosted and cooked through, season and serve. Serves 4, CHO per portion 10g.

DRESSINGS/MISCELLANEOUS

As you have probably realised by now, many of the sauces you buy in the shops contain extra carbohydrates in the form of flour and sugar, as well as other thickeners and preservatives. When you make your own, you can avoid all of these nasties.

For the dressings, we have specified the carbohydrate count for the full recipe, so you can choose how many extra carbohydrates you want to add to your meal with dressings You may be using it for a meal which is low in carbohydrates in general, for example, and you can, therefore, use more of the dressing and vice versa.

Tahini Dressing

This makes a delicious, nutty dressing which you can use for any gutsy salad. It will keep in the fridge for roughly a week. Tahini (crushed sesame seeds) is available in health food shops. We've specified dark tahini, but you can use light if that is all you can find.

1. 8tbsp dark tahini
2. 1tbsp freshly squeezed lemon juice
3. 2tbsp white wine vinegar
4. Salt and freshly-ground black pepper
5. 1tsp garlic puree

Mix the ingredients together well and use to dress the salad. TOTAL CHO – 15g

Real Mayonnaise

If you make, rather than buy, your own mayonnaise, you can be sure of the oil that is used in the product. Many commercial mayonnaises use cheap, refined vegetable oils which can cause inflammation in the body thanks to their high levels of Omega 6s, and non-free-range eggs. Real mayonnaise will not last nearly as long as commercial mayonnaise (a few days in the fridge) so make good plans for it before you make it to avoid waste.

This recipe is much easier if you have a food processor or an electric hand mixer. Otherwise, you may find that whisking it by hand makes a significant contribution to your daily activity levels...

1. 2 egg yolks
2. 1tsp whole grain mustard
3. 250ml olive oil (not the extra virgin kind, which will be too strong)
4. 1tbsp white wine vinegar
5. Salt and white pepper

Place the egg yolks in a bowl with the mustard and whisk well until combined and pale yellow in colour. Add a tiny amount of oil (about a teaspoon) and whisk until well incorporated. Keep adding the oil, a scant teaspoon at a time, until you have added about a quarter of it. You can then start to add the oil in a steady trickle, but be careful – if you add it too quickly, the mixture will curdle.

Once the oil is added, add the vinegar, salt and pepper. (We have suggested white pepper because it's more aesthetically pleasing, but you can use black pepper if you wish).

Additional flavouring ideas: to make it garlicky, add half a clove of garlic, crushed to the final mix and leave for half an hour before serving. To make it herby, finely chop 2tbsp of basil and one tbsp of parsley and mix in. TOTAL CHO – 2g

Stock

Proper stock is the secret to epic gravy (no, it really isn't that plastic-y stuff which begins with a 'B'). You can also add a little salt and drink it as it is as stock contains plenty of vitamins from the vegetables and minerals from the bones.

We have suggested a whole chicken carcass, but you can gather together bones from thighs and legs, for example, when you eat them and store them in the freezer until you have a decent quantity.

1. 1 chicken carcass, stripped off meat
2. 4 large carrots, peeled and roughly chopped (no need to peel if you are using organic carrots)
3. 2 large onions, peeled and roughly chopped
4. 6 cloves garlic, peeled and squashed a little
5. 2tbsp cider vinegar
6. 4 sticks celery, roughly chopped

Place the chicken carcass in a large saucepan/stock pan. Add the veg, garlic and vinegar. Top the pan with water so that everything is well submerged. Place the pan on the hob, cover and heat gently.

Once it has reached a gentle simmer, turn the heat down to its lowest setting and leave for four or five hours. You may need to top up the water levels from time to time, but the longer you can leave the stock (up to 16 hours), the more nutritious it will be as the minerals come off the bones.

Strain and use for gravy and soups. You can also freeze in individual portions.

This recipe is also great made in a slow cooker. Place the ingredients in a slow cooker, top with water, and put on the cooker's lowest setting and leave for 12 hours.

It is almost impossible to calculate the carb content of home-made stock, as the vegetables are strained off the finished product. We think it is negligible.

Low-Carb Gravy

As we said above, the secret of great gravy does not begin with a 'B', it starts with home-made stock. Gravy adapts according to the meat juices you are working with, so we use chicken stock for all gravies as that is the most convenient stock to make, but add the flavour from whatever meat we are cooking with.

1. Pan juices and fat (from your chicken, or other roasted meat)
2. 300ml fresh stock
3. 50ml white wine (use red wine for lamb or beef)
4. 2tbsp double cream (optional)
5. Salt and freshly-ground black pepper

Either use your meat roasting pan with its juices (you can tip off some of the fat, so the gravy isn't too greasy) or tip them into a saucepan.

Add the wine to the pan and bring to the boil, scraping your spoon or whisk around the bottom of the pan to make sure all of the juices and meat flavour is included in the gravy. Once the wine has mostly evaporated, add the stock. Bring to the boil and allow to bubble and reduce by about a third.

This will make a thin gravy so if you want a thicker offering, add the double cream, bring back to the boil and allow to simmer for a few minutes. Add plenty of seasoning and serve. TOTAL CHO – 5g

DESSERTS AND BAKING

Aha – you thought puddings were off the menu now that you have embraced the low-carbohydrate lifestyle? Not so. From time to time, a little sweet treat is necessary, so we've come up with a small selection of recipes which taste delicious, but which stack up far fewer carbohydrates than their conventional versions.

One of the side effects of a low-carbohydrate diet can be, however, the loss of a sweet tooth and you may find yourself satisfied with limited quantities of fruit for a sweet hit. If fruit isn't always hitting the spot though, here are some pudding ideas...

Crème Brulee

1. 4 egg yolks

2. 1/3 cup or 80g or scant 3oz caster sugar (you can use 2/3 of 1/3 cup mixture of Xylitol and Splenda or 2/3 cup Z sweet)

3. 270mls/10 fl oz/1 cup double cream

4. 1 teaspoon each cup for sprinkling REAL sugar on the top once cooked.

Heat oven to 150 degrees/300 degrees F/gas 2 and line a deep baking /roasting tray with grease-proof paper or long-life silicon tray liner.

Whisk the egg yolks and sugar/substitute. Heat the cream in a saucepan until warm but not boiling. Pour it over the egg/sugar mix and put in ramekins.

Put these in the baking tray, and half fill the tray with hot water. Bake in the oven for 35-50 mins. They should wobble just a bit once cooked.

Preheat your grill to its highest setting. Sprinkle the real sugar on top of the custards. Put under the grill until this melts. (You can also use a cook's blow torch to do this job).

Wait a few minutes till the top solidifies and then serve. Serves 4. CHO per portion 10g

Peanut choc chip cookies

1. 125g/4.5oz of chunky peanut butter
2. 185mls/6floz of double cream
3. 75g/2oz chopped pecans or peanuts
4. 35g/1oz chocolate drops or chunks
5. 2 teaspoons vanilla essence
6. 2 tablespoons of granular sugar substitute (see notes below)
7. 2 tablespoons soy flour or coconut flour
8. 1 teaspoon baking powder

Preheat the oven to 190 degrees C/375 degrees F/gas 5 and grease a baking tray or use a silicone liner on a baking tray.

Mix all the ingredients together in a mixer or by hand in a bowl, but put the nuts and choc chips in last.

Put teaspoons of the cookie mixture on the tray and bake for 10 minutes.

These biscuits are very crumbly. Store them in a biscuit tin in the fridge and place layers of kitchen towel between each layer of biscuits. Like a lot of low carb baking, they will last a long time in the fridge, two to three weeks.

If you double the recipe up, as you may well do, the amount of peanut butter is just short of a jar. Just use up the whole jar. It doesn't matter.

Don't try to make your own chocolate chunks. I destroyed a mini chopper doing this.

You can either use straight Splenda or in place of one tablespoon of Splenda ¼ tablespoon Splenda and ½ tablespoon of xylitol or erythritol. Another substitute is 1/3 tablespoon of Truvia.

Sponge Cake and Variations *(contributed by Fergus Craig)*

Low Carb Sponge Cake (makes one layer)

1. 85g butter
2. 2 tablespoons olive oil
3. 3 eggs
4. 200g ground almonds
5. 1tsp baking powder
6. 1tbsp your choice of granular sugar substitute (see peanut choc/chip cookies for options)

Preheat oven to 170 C. Cream the butter and sweetener until light and fluffy, Add the olive oil and eggs and mix well, then add the almonds and baking powder.

Pour into a greased, lined 20-cm cake tin or springform cake tin and bake for 30 minutes.

If you are making a Victoria sponge, you will need to make two cakes. Just double the recipe and bake for the same time. This recipe also works as a base for Tiramisu and for a chocolate sponge cake. You would simply add a heaped tablespoon of cocoa per cake.

To make a low-carb trifle:

Cut the cake up and put it at the bottom of your best big glass bowl. Then pour some alcoholic liquor over it. Sherry is traditional, but there are other things you can use such as brandy and other liqueurs.

You can use commercial low carb jelly, either raspberry or strawberry in the recipe. This is optional. Make it up with hot water and then pour over the boozy sponge.

Add some fruit of your choice. Raspberries work the best as they are low in carbohydrate. Other items could be chopped tinned apricots or pears.

If you are using jelly, put in the fridge until set.

A perfect cheat's custard to go on top of this is to use 250g mascarpone mixed with a dessert spoon of granular sugar substitute and 2 egg yolks. You may also add brandy or sherry to this too. Whisk the egg whites separately till stiff and fold in.

Put your boozy trifle in the fridge and eat after one hour or more.

Victoria Sponge

Make two of the sponge cakes. Spread one with 2 tablespoons sugar reduced raspberry jam and whipped cream. Put the cake with the evenest top on the top.

Chocolate Sponge

Make the cakes as described but add the cocoa before baking. Layer with whipped cream.

Tiramisu

You can use either the plain or chocolate sponges for this dish. You will need one sponge cake, but you may not need all of it. It depends on the size of your bowl.

Cut the sponge into strips to fit a nice glass bowl. Soak the sponge in any of these: Tia Maria, Kahlua, Rum, or Amaretto.

For the creamy filling, separate six eggs. Beat the yolks with about three heaped tablespoons of granular sugar substitute. (Try 2 tbsp Xylitol and 1 tbsp Splenda). Add 500g mascarpone and some Amaretto or Kahlua or Tia Maria. Whip together.

In a jug, put 250mls of cooled strong coffee (preferably real) and ¼ cup brandy or Kahlua or Tia Maria.

Whip the egg whites and once stiff, fold them into the boozy/cheese mixture.

Using your nicest bowl, put in a layer of sponge cut up. Dribble over the coffee mixture until the sponge is wet but not disintegrating.

Add a good layer of boozy custard. Keep on going till you have a layer of boozy custard on top. Put chocolate shavings or cocoa powder on top. Put it in the fridge for at least two hours before serving to chill.

This keeps for a few days if you can keep your hands off it. Serves 4. CHO per portion 15g

Cherry Frangipane Tart

This is a gorgeous buttery pudding that can do well at breakfast.

1. 2 cups ground almonds (200g)
2. 1 cup whey protein powder plain or vanilla
3. 3 tablespoons granular sugar substitute
4. One teaspoon ground cinnamon
5. 200g very soft unsalted butter

Preheat the oven to 210 C degrees. Stick all the ingredients in your food mixer. When it is a soft dough, take it out and form it into a pie crust. This amount is enough to cover the bottom and sides of a 12-inch base with 2-inch sides.

Put this in an oven for five minutes then take it out. Turn down the oven to 180 degrees. Meanwhile, mix up the frangipane and fruit filling:

1. 200g very soft unsalted butter
2. 1 cup granular sugar substitute (or use my formula which is: ½ cup Xylitol and ¼ cup Splenda)
3. 2 eggs
4. 200g ground almonds

Stick all this in your food mixer and blend together. Put this inside the cooked or at least partially cooked tart.

Cut up a big handful of cherries into halves and remove the stones. Place these on top of the frangipane in a nice pattern. You can also use ripe plums or improvise with what fruit you have, such as pears and apricots.

Scatter one teaspoon of real caster sugar on top of the fruit on the pie. This gives a superior caramelisation effect to the pie which sugar substitutes can't match.

Stick this in the oven for one hour. After this time, check on the pie every ten minutes to see if it is wobbly in the middle. Once it wobbles only very slightly, turn off the oven and let it cool. It is easiest to portion out the pie before it becomes cold and stiff from refrigeration. After that, the pie is best heated in the microwave or oven before eating.

Serve with cream.

Apple pie

You can make a delicious low carb/wheat free apple pie with a lid. This is how.

Take eight eating apples, peel and chop them roughly. Put them in a small quantity of water in a saucepan and bring to the boil. Simmer until tender. You may add a small amount of granular sugar substitute or liquid Stevia to taste.

Make up the low-carb pastry but add a third again, so you have enough pastry for a lid.

The quantities are thus:

1. 3 cups ground almonds (300g)
2. 1½ cups whey protein powder plain or vanilla
3. 4 tablespoons granular sugar substitute
4. One heaped teaspoon ground cinnamon
5. 300g very soft unsalted butter

Stick all of the ingredients in your food mixer. When a soft dough has formed, take it out and divide into three equal-sized balls. You will use one for the base, one for the sides and one for the lid.

Push the base pastry ball into the bottom and spread on your 12-inch diameter pie pan. Take smaller amounts of the next ball of dough and press them into the sides until it goes all the way round. Now add the cooked apples.

The tricky part is putting on the lid. Because this dough is so soft and has none of the elasticity of a wheat dough, you can't roll it out like "normal" pastry and pop the lid on the top.

You need to get some silicon sheet or parchment paper. Roll the remainder of the pastry in your hand till it is in a ball shape. Put it in the middle of your silicon sheet and roll it out in a circle. You will use whey protein powder to reduce sticking just as you would flour in traditional pastry making. It is best to handle the dough as little as possible.

Make a circle slightly bigger than the diameter of the pie top. This is the tricky part! As quickly and accurately as you can, place the pastry lid on top of the pie. Now peel off the silicon paper on top. If you have missed a bit, you will have some pastry left over at the opposite end of the pie, so cut this off and do some repair work till the pie top is complete. Cut two slots on the top of the pie so air can escape.

Put this in an oven at 210 degrees for 5 minutes then turn down the oven to 180 degrees and cook for approximately 20 minutes till the crust is golden. Serve with low carb custard (see trifle recipe) or double cream. Keeps well in the fridge for a few days but is at its best on the day of cooking. Serves 8, CHO per portion – 20g.

Don't forget – we have hundreds of recipes online at the Diabetes Diet website – https://diabetesdietblog.com

CHAPTER 11

HOW TO EXERCISE WITH DIABETES

This might be the section in the book that you may well wish to skip, but bear with us while we explain why it's good for people with diabetes to exercise and how you can fit it into your life.

Exercise isn't just about huffing and puffing in the gym, something many people find off-putting. Think of it, instead, as a way of incorporating more activity into your life and it will seem much friendlier and more do-able!

We may not agree with the dietary recommendations of various governmental and health organisations in the US and the UK, but we DO agree with them about exercise. Thanks to modern lifestyles, changes in the way we work and the way we travel to work, large swathes of the population are much less physically active than they were in the earlier part of the 20th century and even up until the 1960s/1970s.

The latter part of the 20th century saw an explosion in the car-owning population, a tremendous growth in office-based sedentary jobs and numerous labour-saving devices which robbed us of the chance of taking exercise – escalators, lifts, remote controls, sit on lawnmowers, washing machines... You name it, there's some automated way you can save yourself from moving.

There are easy ways to add activity to your life – not just exercise which involves pulling on gym gear and sweating it out on a treadmill or in a class – which we will go in to later, but firstly what are the advantages to exercising or activity when you have diabetes?

In this book, we are keen that you get the idea that looking after yourself is YOUR job and not your doctor's, and, to quote from Mr Motivator Derrick Evans, *"Exercise is the best life insurance you can take out"*. Hear, hear!

Eat properly and add in exercise to your life, because exercise and activity act as an anti-ageing cure across the board.

So why is it important for diabetics to exercise or incorporate regular activity? A well-balanced exercise or activity plan (which includes a cardio, strength and flexibility element) will have several benefits. It will:

1. increase the body's sensitivity to insulin

2. lower blood-sugar levels

3. lower blood pressure

4. increase fat loss

5. build muscle mass

6. reduce stress

7. improve circulation.

Reduced sensitivity to insulin, high blood sugar levels, high blood pressure, elevated levels of body fat and bad circulation are side effects of type 2 diabetes and poorly controlled type 1 diabetes, which is where exercise can help. Insulin resistance is, in fact, lowered to a greater extent by weight training, rather than other forms of exercise.

It can also reduce stress and improve your mood. The lowering of blood sugar, blood pressure etc. are probably benefits for diabetics you could have guessed at, but what about some of the less obvious advantages?

With a well-designed strength and stretching programme (accompanied of course by our low-carbohydrate eating plan), you can build more muscle mass and decrease the amount of body fat you have. Not only is this aesthetically pleasing (a slender, toned body has more to do with lower body fat levels than actual body weight), but more muscle mass means greater sensitivity to insulin – great for preventing diabetes, but if you already have diabetes you can decrease how much insulin you need to take.

A more muscular frame can allow you to eat a little more, as your metabolic rate is dependent to some extent on your muscularity.

Bone density is worse in people with diabetes so this can increase the risk of falls which result in fractured bones. Weight-bearing exercise, such as walking, running or lifting weights, can increase bone density, while exercises which test our balance can improve balance and decrease the risk of falling.

Lack of flexibility is another diabetes risk. Diabetics tend to get stiffness in tendons due to the glycation of collagen, which significantly worsens the stiffening effects that are seen in normal ageing. To avoid it, practise stretching exercises on a regular, if not daily, basis.

EXERCISE AND LOWERED BLOOD SUGAR LEVELS

As the benefits of exercise outlined at the beginning show, reduced blood sugar levels is one excellent reason to exercise, but what about the risk of hypoglycaemia, where blood sugars go too low?

If you are taking insulin or a blood-sugar lowering medication, then exercise can lower blood sugar levels – it depends on a number of factors:

1. What your blood sugar was before starting

2. What time of day it is

3. What you last ate

4. What time of the month it is (for women of menstruating age only)

5. How intense your exercise session is

6. How long your training session lasts

Obviously, the more intense or the longer-lasting your exercise session is, the more likely you are to have a hypo. [Although just to be awkward, this isn't always the case. See the note on exercising with high blood sugars in the FAQs section.]

Depending on how your blood sugar see-saws around during the day will also affect your body. If for example, your blood sugar tends to rise in the mornings then exercise can sometimes counteract this effect, or at least mean the activity at this time of the day will not affect your blood sugar levels.

Again, if you are planning an intense, or long-lasting session and you do not eat something with carbohydrates in it before exercising, then hypos are a risk.

If you are a woman of menstruating age, you are likely to suffer insulin resistance in the week or so before your period is due, which means your blood sugar levels run high and makes you less likely to experience a hypo when exercising at this time.

If your blood sugar level is below a certain threshold before you start (and this varies from individual to individual, and depends on the kind of exercise being undertaken), then you are more likely to experience a hypo.

The answer, we're afraid to say, isn't simple. It depends on a whole lot of different factors, and it varies widely between individuals. You will need to work this out for yourself by doing lots of blood tests before, during and after exercise. If your activity is different on one day, then the medications and additional food regime which worked for you for one activity may not work for a different one.

Exercise can have an effect on our bodies hours after we exercise, so that is also something to bear in mind as you may need to adjust your medications hours afterwards as well.

It goes without saying that the exercising diabetic who is using insulin should carry fast-acting glucose with them and make sure that anyone who is with them knows they have diabetes. Explain the symptoms of your hypos to them too.

Finally, the list of variations to be taken into consideration can make exercise look daunting. Routine is something, however, that works well for people with diabetes. If you exercise regularly, your body will get used to exercise and adapt. The first time you attempt a run may leave you experiencing low blood sugars afterwards and not just one of them, but perhaps a few of them over 24 hours. Once your body has got fitter and used to the routine, the risk of hypos decreases.

So, what are the components of a well-rounded exercise routine? As we said before, cardio, strength and flexibility are the three pillars of fitness.

There are, however, some limits to what people with diabetes complications can do so read on to gain a full understanding of exercise, its benefits and what you should or should not do.

Let's start with psychological limits which apply to everyone and not just those with diabetes – the inclination to exercise. The main factors that people say limit the amount of activity they do are not having the time, and not having the inclination.

As we said before, those of us living in the modern western world live in a society set up for minimal exercise. You can quite easily do nothing, as many jobs are sedentary. Most people either travel to work by car, bus or train and our leisure time often involves sitting down activities – watching TV, going to the cinema, meeting friends for coffee/drinks/food, sunbathing on holiday and so forth – so often the exercise thing needs to be forced.

A modern phenomenon, the active couch potato, tells of people who otherwise lead sedentary daily lives but who haul themselves off to the gym or a class five or six days a week and think they are counteracting the 23 hours out of 24 daily inactivity. Studies have shown this not to be the case[111]. So, the first thing to do is look at your day as a whole and work out where you can squeeze in anything which involves moving and walking around, instead of sitting.

We'll cover ideas for daily "non-exercise" activity at the end of this chapter, but for the meantime, here are some motivational ideas for those of you who DO want to follow a more formalised exercise plan:

Make a bargain with yourself that you will do 10 minutes of exercise/activity a day. If you start small, you are more likely to keep it up. Exercise is great for boosting your mood, and the chances are that after the first 10-minute block, you will feel good and you may well wish to continue.

Find activities you can do in front of the TV or that fit in with your daily life. Lifting weights or performing bodyweight exercises while watching TV in the evening can work this way, just as choosing to walk or cycle to the shops instead of taking the car for short journeys can take the same amount of time.

Find an exercise buddy. It is easy to let yourself down by not exercising, but harder to let someone else down. A friend to go walking with can make the experience much more enjoyable.

Exercise straight after work. If you think of exercise as part of your working day (and therefore non-negotiable), then you can get into a routine of always exercising after work and then having the rest of your evening to yourself. Having to come home and then go straight back out again to the gym or a class can make it easier to abandon the exercise idea altogether.

Get into your exercise gear as soon as you get up or come home – you are more likely to exercise if you are dressed in the proper gear.

Avoid sitting down in front of your computer if you are intending to exercise. It's too easy to get distracted.

You may not be fit enough to exercise for 40 minutes to an hour to start with, but everyone has 10 minutes. We recommend you start with this till you get into the exercise habit.

It has been found that exercise of 10-minute segments throughout the day is as good as doing a session of exercise all at once. Use this to your advantage.

Cardiovascular Fitness

Anything that gets your heart pumping faster and gets you sweaty is improving your cardiovascular fitness to some extent. Cardiovascular fitness is important because while carrying it out, your heart and lungs need to work harder to supply your body with enough oxygen for fuel. Exercised lungs and hearts are more efficient and healthier.

An excellent example of cardio exercise is walking, and this is suitable for ALL diabetics. Walk at a pace that is brisk and includes hills if you can. Running or jogging is another cardio exercise, but best done by those who are already fit and people who have proliferative retinopathy (damage to the eyes) should not do it to avoid further blood vessel damage.

In the gym, you can use exercise bikes, Nordic tracks, rowing machines and treadmills to get your heart rate up.

To make your exercise more sociable, ballroom and other kinds of dancing are good fun. If you are a gym-phobe, then you might prefer outdoor activities such as hill walking, orienteering, horse riding or golf.

Those who relish competition can join in with sports such as tennis, badminton and football (do ensure you warm up properly first).

To get really fit, you can try interval training which alternates cardio work with a less intense or different form of activity, such as running followed by walking, or jumping jacks interspersed with muscle-building activity, or running up hills and then walking down to recover.

High-intensity interval training (where you work as hard as you can for a short period such as 30 seconds or a minute, rest for a short period and then start again) needs a good level of fitness to start with because there is less recovery between the high-impact moves and the lower intensity moves.

However, HIIT is thought to be very, very good for our hearts and a 10-minute HIIT session (one-minute fast sprints on an exercise bike with one-minute rest in between) three times a week provides the same fitness results as 10 hours of steady cycling over a two-week period[112].

Please note – if you have type 1 diabetes, HIIT can put your blood sugar up alarmingly. Check your blood sugars afterwards. You might need to take a small amount of insulin to correct.

All these activities tend to build cardio–vascular endurance so it becomes progressively easier to do the activities or extend the time or the pace that you can do them.

Getting Started: Basic Aerobic Exercise

To start an aerobic exercise programme, start by walking for five minutes a day away from your house as briskly as you can and walking back at a gentler pace.

Increase this gradually to one hour a day. You can also do shorter walks several times a day if that is easier to fit in. You may add longer weekend walks into your total.

All diabetics should be able to do this. Make sure your socks and shoes are well fitting and comfortable. If you have neuropathy (nerve damage) check the linings are smooth before putting them on.

Strength

Weight training can be done by everyone. It is more important the older you are because we lose muscle mass as we get older and more muscle mass is important because it increases insulin sensitivity.

Many strength routines also have a cardiac training effect because your heart rate is elevated over 120 beats per minute, especially during kettlebells and weight training. In some cases, a strength routine can push the heart rate up to higher levels than so-called cardio activities.

Kettlebell exercises improve strength and cardiovascular fitness. Resistance bands are easily portable and come in different strengths. You pull against the band, and this strengthens the muscle.

Body weight exercises can be done with no equipment in your living room.

Getting Started: Basic Strength Exercises

An effective strength routine can incorporate cardiac training too, so prioritise strength training if you can.

You can start strength training with bodyweight exercises, practised every second day. Do them in front of your TV if that helps as an incentive. Warm up with five minutes of jogging on the spot, jumping jacks, hip circles, arm circles and knee circles.

1. Press-ups
2. Squats
3. The plank
4. Tricep dips
5. Lunges

6. Backward lunges

7. Wall sit

8. V sit

9. Russian twists

10. Calf raises

11. Back extensions

12. Bottom/hamstring squeezes

Press-ups – With your knees on the floor (use a cushion for comfort), put your forearms out in front of you and have your arms wider than your chest. Go up and down slowly. Once you can do three sets of 8 increase the challenge by doing press ups on your toes.

Squats – Standing up with your legs about shoulder-width apart, stick your bottom out and lower it as if you are going to sit on a chair. When your legs are at right angles (you may not be able to get as low as this at first), stand up slowly and squeeze your buttock muscles as you do.

The plank – kneel on the floor. Put both hands out in front of you at shoulder level and push up to your knees. Hold this for 20 seconds and build up gradually to one minute. When you can do this, go up to your toes, hold for 20 seconds and build that up to a minute as well.

Tricep dips – using a dining chair or coffee table, sit close to the edge with your hands facing forward flat on the surface. Move forward so that your bottom is unsupported from the edge and use your arms to lower your bottom and pushing up again. Keep your elbows facing backwards at all times. Perform three sets of 8. To make the exercise easier, you can do it on the floor with your arms behind. To make it more challenging, you can straighten out your legs while on the chair, or cross one leg over the other.

Lunges – stand with your feet just over hip width apart. Take a step forward with one leg and hold your torso upright. Bend your legs and bring your bottom down until your knees are at 90 degrees. Squeeze your legs as you come back up. For backward lunges, take the leg behind you and perform in the same way.

Wall sit – stand with your back against a wall with your feet shoulder-width apart. Slide down the wall slowly until your legs are roughly at right angles to the wall. Hold the position for 20 seconds and do this three times. Build up slowly to 45-60 seconds.

V sit – sit on the floor and lift your legs off the floor. Lean back slowly until your body is in a V position and hold the position for 20 seconds. Do this three times and build up slowly to 45-60 seconds.

Russian twist – sitting in a v-sit position, cross your ankles and twist your body from side to side, touching the floor each side as you do so. Aim for 10 touches each side.

Calf raises – standing with your feet shoulder-width apart, lift your heels off the floor slowly and then drop them back to the floor. Repeat for three sets of 8. (This is an old ballet exercise and ballerinas regularly did this one for 100 repeats. You can build up to that if you want, but we must warn that it BURNS.)

Back extensions – lying face down on the floor, place your hands under your chin and slowly raise your torso off the floor. Hold for a couple of seconds at the top. Do this for three sets of eight.

Bottom/hamstring squeezes – lie on your back, arms by your sides. Place your knees on the floor away from your bottom hip-width apart. Raise your bottom off the floor and squeeze your buttocks and hamstrings. You can make this harder by putting one leg over the other thigh to give extra weight or holding one leg at the level of the knee of the moving leg.

We know this looks like a lot of exercise, but it should not take too long. If you are really pushed, pick out five or six exercises ensuring you have ones that work the upper body, the lower body and the stomach.

For a detailed strength routine with weights and a quick warm-up routine, see appendices A and B.

Flexibility

Flexibility tends to take time to develop. People who work in offices or who spend large parts of their day sitting can be very inflexible, and that inflexibility can have built up over many years, if not decades.

For the best effects, you need to hold a stretch for 45 seconds. Examples of exercise routines which include a lot of stretching of muscles such as:

1. Athletic stretching exercises
2. Yoga
3. Ballet dancing
4. Barre exercises
5. Pilates.

Balance

As we discussed before, balance is necessary to decrease the risk of falls (and possibilities of fractured bones). You can improve your balance at any age by practising. To start with, hold onto the back of a chair to help until your balance improves.

Balance moves are included in Wii fitness games, dance, yoga and Pilates.

Coordination

Coordination can worsen as we age. To improve it, it is easier to start with athletic moves which require less coordination than dance type moves.

If you want to improve your coordination, look for sporting activities which stress hand to eye coordination (racquet and ball games), Wii fitness games and dance.

Getting Started – Basic Stretch Routine

You start this routine standing and then move to the floor as you get nearer the end. Hold all stretches for 45 seconds. Put on some music you like (or the TV) and time the stretches.

Neck stretch – stand upright with your legs hip width apart. Place one arm behind your back. Put the other on the top of your head and gently ease your head towards your shoulder. Repeat on the other side.

Triceps stretch – raise one arm in the air beside your head and bend the arm. Pull on your elbow gently to stretch the triceps muscle of the raised arm. Repeat on the other side.

Shoulder stretch – put one arm out in front of you. Now take it directly across your chest at shoulder level and gently pull on it above elbow level with the other hand so that you feel a stretch at the shoulder. Repeat on the other side.

Chest stretch – stand with your feet shoulder-width apart and clasp your hands behind you, keeping them as straight as possible and with your palms facing into your back. Raise your arms until you feel the stretch across your chest.

Back stretch – stand with your legs shoulder width apart. Bend your knees. Clasp your hands under your knees and vary the position till you feel a stretch in different parts of the back as you pull with both hands with your spine curved.

Reach up – raise the arms in the air and gently stretch one arm up and then the other feeling the stretch in your abdomen, the sides of the body, shoulders and arms.

Calf stretch – take one leg behind you and place your hands on your hip. Lean forward so that your front leg bends and feel the stretch along the calf of the back leg. Repeat on the other side.

Butterfly stretch – sit up with the soles of both feet touching each other and your elbows on your knees, hands clasped. Bend your torso forward till you feel the stretch in your inner thighs and push your thighs as flat to the floor as you can get them.

Quadriceps – lie on one side with the lower leg bent and your elbow on the ground. Use your other hand to pull on your foot so that you get a stretch down the quadriceps of the upper leg. Repeat on the other side.

Alternating types of workout

There is no reason why you can't do cardio exercises or stretching exercises every day. Weight training, however, is best done once or twice a week if you use hefty weights and no more than alternate days if you are using light weights or your body weight.

The idea with weight training is that you will gradually increase the weights as you go along, moving from bodyweight exercises to light weights and eventually heavy weights.

For this reason, it is best that you plan your weight training days in advance and fill in the other days with walking and/or stretching.

Stretching can be done on its own but is also beneficial after a session of walking or weight training.

It is common to feel muscle soreness the day after an exercise session that has challenged you. This is the point! It can persist for a few days.

Here is a sample workout plan based on a period of three weeks:

1. heavy weight training
2. abs and back exercises
3. walk in the country
4. heavy weight training
5. abs and stretch
6. Badminton
7. heavy weight training
8. abs and cardio
9. Dancing
10. heavy weight training
11. yoga
12. easy toning/cardio
13. cardio
14. heavy weight training
15. rowing + meditation/relaxation
16. easy toning/cardio
17. abs + Wii fitness games
18. kettlebell
19. aerobics and yoga
20. kettlebell
21. walk and stretch

Remember, this is a sample for someone used to exercise. Start slowly and build up to whatever you can do. You can create your own training rota, perhaps based on what days of the week are most suitable for different activities. A walk outside is probably more fun in daylight and good weather for instance.

High Blood Sugar Levels and Exercise

Just as low blood sugar levels can stop you exercising, so can high ones. If your blood sugar level is 11mmol (191mg) or above before you start to exercise, then exercise is going to be extremely difficult.

The body reacts to the tiredness of high blood sugars by trying to pull glucose out of the muscles to compensate – sending your blood sugar levels even higher. Yikes!

You will feel as if you are wading through the thickest, blackest, stickiest treacle and it's no fun at all.

You can fix this by giving a short dose of insulin 15-30 minutes before you are due to start exercising – give yourself about half the dose you would usually need to lower your blood sugar, as once you start exercising the insulin and the exercise will work together.

"Non-Exercise" Activities

In days of old, there was no such thing as aerobics, spin classes and weights rooms. You were fit thanks to your daily activities. If the thought of the gym or being barked at by a Lycra-clad lovely are a real turn off, why not look to other activities to increase your heart rate?

1. Walking out and back – see our recommendation in the basic cardiovascular fitness section.

2. Resolving to walk, instead of taking the car for all short journeys.

3. Heavy housework – polishing, vacuum cleaning, scrubbing shelves, changing beds and others can work up a slight sweat if done vigorously enough. Do them on a regular basis, though.

4. Dancing to songs on the radio – 10-minute bursts of energetic dancing will make you feel hot and invigorated. Use your own playlist if you can't find anything you like.

5. Never use the elevators or lifts in buildings if you can avoid it. Regular stair-climbing is great for heart health.

6. Standing up wherever you can. Sitting down for long periods does no-one any favours. If you do an office-based job or you sit in front of computers for an extended period of time, resolve to get up and go for a short walk around every hour. You can even look into standing desks for computers, or stand up to make phone calls just so that you aren't sitting for such long periods of time.

Our Experiences

Dr Morrison – time is one of the reasons many people give for not exercising, which is understandable in modern life. I work as a doctor and, although I work more reasonable hours now, I previously worked 100 hours or more a week.

When I started to do regular exercise at the age of 25, I was incredibly unfit. Long hours studying and working had had their effect. I could not walk up two flights of stairs without becoming breathless. I realised I was about as fit as most 80-year-olds and, once my working schedule allowed, I started to go to classes through the week and hill walking and then skiing at weekends.

Once I became a GP and police surgeon, I joined a gym and went two or three times a week. I also went swimming once a week in addition to walking at weekends. There were aerobic classes run by physiotherapists at the hospital, and I went once a week. I went to yoga a few times but found it impossible. I was so stiff I could hardly do any poses, and the balance exercises were beyond me.

My starting weight at the gym for arm exercises was 0.5kg, and I did 20 reps...

After being a gym member for three years, the price went up, so I went to WH Smith to buy a Kathy Smith exercise DVD. I started doing this 15 minutes a day in my living room after work every day.

Home exercise videos, DVDs and the Wii have become my preferred method of routine exercise. You can do them any time that suits. I have about 350 DVDs/videos. I also walk with friends regularly and swim when I am on holiday.

If I waited till I had done everything I needed before leaving the house in the mornings, or waited till I have had my dinner or when I come home from work at night, I know that I would not manage to exercise daily. What suits me is a form of interval training that incorporates home exercise with self-care and housework.

A typical morning routine alternates 10-minute exercise with taking pills, putting on make-up, cleaning the kitchen, and finally having a tea break during which I pay bills, make phone calls or respond to emails.

It can be quite a challenge to work out when it is a cold, dark, and dreich outside. The best option I have found is to put on DVDs where the presenter is in a sunny outside location, and you can pretend you are working out with your imaginary friends in the sun.

Emma Baird – I have been exercising since my teens, although I do go through fits and starts with it. I'm also a bit of a fitness tart and change my allegiance on a frequent basis.

I have, therefore, tried every fitness craze going – from the gym, to spin classes, to running, to walking, to Callanetics, exercise DVDs, Pilates, personal trainers, Bikram yoga, body pump, tae bo, power plates, aqua aerobics and more...

These days, like the good doctor, I do like exercise DVDs for their convenience. You can do them whenever suits and, if you are in your grottiest gym gear which honestly should have been in the wash days ago, it doesn't matter.

I have stuck to walking, Pilates, and body weight/weights routines over the years though too.

CHAPTER 12

USEFUL TOOLS FOR GETTING STARTED ON LOW-CARBING AND RECOMMENDED READING

Here are some of the tools we recommend for getting started on a low-carbohydrate diet plan:

Our blog: http://diabetesdietblog.com contains even more news, information, tips and recipes.

Digital kitchen scales – they can help you measure foods precisely. A set of proper measuring tablespoons and teaspoons is useful too, as well as a set of cups as many low-carb recipes use cup measurements. A Tala measuring cup gives both UK and USA cup measurements and gives volume based weights for many dry ingredients.

A carbohydrate counting book – Collins produces a comprehensive small guide which you can keep in the house or in your handbag. There are also plentiful online resources such as:

- www.myfitnesspal.com
- http://www.fitday.com/

You can also get a free carb counting guide from:

http://www.diabetes.org.uk/Guide-to-diabetes/Managing-your-diabetes/Carb-counting/

For books on diabetes and low-carbohydrate dieting, see:

231

1. Dr Richard Bernstein's Diabetes Solution: A Complete Guide to Achieving Normal Blood Sugars (Little, Brown US; 4th edition)

2. Think Like a Pancreas: A Practical Guide to Managing Diabetes with Insulin by Gary Scheiner (Da Capo Lifelong Books – Second Edition)

3. Dana Carpender's 500 Low-Carb Recipes (Fair Winds) is a comprehensive collection of recipes, although some of the ingredients may not be available in the UK

4. The New High Protein Diet by Dr Charles and Maureen Clark (Vermillion) has a great collection of recipes, as they are easily divided or multiplied, and they use UK measurements.

5. Karen Barnaby's The Low Carb Gourmet (Harper Collins)

6. Robert Atkins' The New Illustrated Low Carb Cookbook (Vermillion)

7. Sharon Long's Extreme Lo-carb Meals on the Go (Adams Media)

For a clinical report on the success of low-carbohydrate diets on people with type 1 diabetes, see:

1. A Low Carbohydrate Diet in Type 1 Diabetes: Clinical Experience – a Brief Report by JV Nielson, E Jonsson and A Ivarsson

2. For lots of information on managing medication, low carbohydrate eating and diabetes, see http://www.dsolve.com/

3. Check out the forums on diabetes.co.uk, as there are plenty of people discussing low-carb dieting here. They also have a low carbohydrate diabetes course.

There are lots of low-carbohydrate diet plans, sample menus and recipe ideas out there online, but many of them are American – so the measurements and ingredients can be unfamiliar, as can American names for different ingredients such as zucchini for courgettes and cilantro for coriander.

However, for great nutritional advice and samples plans, check out Authority Nutrition, a really informative website about low-carbohydrate eating with the added bonus that the author isn't permanently trying to flog you something...

As you know, we like exercise DVDs for their variety and versatility. Here are some personal recommendations:

Cardio and Strength:

1. Davina McCall's exercise DVDs are comprehensive and include good cardio/strength training sections which are well explained.

2. Jillian Michaels also produces excellent DVDs. We like 30 Day Shred (though the weight loss claims that come with it are to be taken with a pinch of salt).

3. Mr Motivator's 10-minute Work-outs can easily be fitted into your day

4. Jane Fonda's Workout with Weights

5. Reinhardt Kettlebell System

6. Lorraine Kelly Pink and Green workouts

7. Ada Jankowitz Basic Training

8. Gilad Jankowitz Cuts and Curves and Lord of the Abs (ball) workouts

9. Karen Voight: Arms and Abs

10. Kathy Smith: Ultimate stomach, thighs and bums workout and Secrets of a Great Body Upper and Lower workouts

11. Jessica Smith 10 minute solution Quick Tummy Toners

12. Chalean Extreme weight workout set

13. Tamilee Web Tight on Time workouts

14. Tracey Staehle The Parts workout

15. Angie Miller: Kettlebell Bootcamp, Core strength and fusion, Crave results, and Bedroom body workouts.

16. Kelly Coffee Meyer: Muscle Definition and Split Sessions

17. Jari Love: Ripped to the Core and Rev'd to the Max Workouts

18. Cathe Freidrich: Slow and Heavy and many other weight training workouts

Yoga and Relaxation:

1. Leah Bracknell: Yoga for life

2. Rodney Yee: Yoga for relaxation

3. Madeleine Lewis: Am and Pm stretch

4. Scott Cole: Yoga and Tai Chi

5. Bodhipaksa: Mindfulness

There are lots of exercise and fitness DVDs out there – look at reviews to find the one that works for you and check out charity shops to pick them up for a reduced price. You can also swap with friends.

You can also download apps for your phone or tablet. Sworkit Pro has a range of workouts from cardio to yoga, body weight and stretching. You can choose the workout and the duration and mix them up for a varied workout.

My fitness coach on Wii also works well and can be used for any kind of exercise – from cardio to weights to balance.

And, of course, there is YouTube. You could do a work-out for every day of the year on YouTube and never do the same one twice. Look for the ones posted by Bodybuilding.com, Pop Sugar and Joe Wicks (for HIIT).

Please note – these are our personal recommendations, based on our own use. We have received no financial recompense or sponsorship from any of the products.

CONCLUSIONS

Here we are at the end of our book...

We hope you have found it interesting and we hope that you feel as if you have a better understanding of how you can benefit your health and your diabetes control by applying the methods we have suggested. Good health is within your grasp – we promise.

At the time of writing, the number of diabetics worldwide stands at 422 million[113] (and many more people will be undiagnosed). This figure will increase, and bring with it the resultant complications.

YOU have the best possible methods for preventing those conditions and to give you the recipe for a happy, healthy and fulfilled life – despite diabetes.

We know that it can be hard for people to stick to low-carbing in the long term. Many people are addicted to carbohydrates and, like any addiction, it takes considerable effort and retraining of habits to break.

Others find it a great inconvenience to have to plan, shop and cook from scratch. Unpleasant though it may seem to think about, you have to put at the front of your mind what the unpleasantness and inconvenience that not being able to see, not being able to walk and being in constant pain feels like, as unfortunately, this is what awaits if blood sugars are not brought under control.

To get this control you need the correct information about what to do, and then you need to do it consistently. It is certainly a lot easier if you have the support of your family and your medical team.

Many people are initially appalled at the number of blood tests, carb counting and insulin dose recording they have to do to discover exactly how to get the blood sugars they want. When you do not have diabetes, you rely on your pancreas do all of this sophisticated calculation for you. Sadly, you are not in the situation where you can just rely on your pancreas, so the choice of whether or not to do the necessary self-experimentation becomes quite stark.

It does get easier with time. Meanwhile, you need to look at every meal as a scientific experiment on how good you can become at thinking like a pancreas.

Your efforts to guess what you need to do, and then test to see how close you got to your target blood sugars, bring you a step closer every time to mastering your blood sugars and regaining your life.

For those of you who are not on insulin, blood sugar management can be a pretty straightforward process by adopting this approach, especially if you stick to the lower glycaemic vegetables as your main source of carbohydrate.

If you are on insulin, the detailed information we are giving you can seem hopelessly complicated when you first see it. Yet, insulin management is not so much a difficult problem, such as rocket science, and more like a complex issue, such as building a house. There are lots of components and choice points that are there to give you the greatest flexibility.

Should you decide to stick at 30g of carb for each of your main meals without the added complexity of knowing how to titrate your insulin doses up and down for different amounts of carbs at different times of day, this could suit you very well. It is the backbone of the diet recommended for all diabetics by the American Association of Clinical Endocrinologists and has been shown to be very effective in long-term studies on types one and two diabetes carried out by Swedish Diabetologist Dr Jorgen Vesti Nielsen and in expectant and pregnant women by USA Diabetologist Dr Lois Jovanovich.

It will take time and practice to get it right for you. There will be mistakes along the way, and there will be temptation everywhere, but carbohydrate restriction and precise medication matching do get easier as you keep on going with it. Once it becomes a habit, you no longer need to use will power and automatically eating and selecting low-carb choices, turning down bread, and refusing cakes and biscuits will be second nature.

There will be the odd time when you want to eat something higher in carbohydrates. Eat the food mindfully, make it an occasional treat and make sure it is the best possible version of that food – a home-made cake, or pizza made by someone who knows what they are doing, artisan bread or a meal in a good restaurant. Match your insulin as best as you can, go for a walk afterwards and then jump back on the low-carb diet.

We wish you success with the methods we have discussed in our book and a long, complication free and happy life.

Please visit us at https://diabetesdietblog.com/ or email us: lowcarbdiabetesdiet@gmail.com

Dr Katharine Morrison
Emma Baird

ACKNOWLEDGEMENTS
– AND THANKS FOR READING

We hope you have enjoyed our book and found it useful. Do keep in touch with us via our accompanying website, www. diabetesdietblog.com which includes further information, courses, and recipes.

Katharine would like to thank her son Steven who has eaten a multitude of low carb meals and baking over the years. Not all of these turned out that well first go, but he ate them just the same. Also her son David, who suggested she use the "empty nest" as an opportunity to write this book.

The original diabetes course at www.dsolve.com on which this book is based could not have been produced without the help of the pioneering work of Dr Richard Bernstein and members of his forum, particularly Ryan Whitaker.

The help and support of the members of the Nutrition and Metabolism Society particularly Professor Richard Feinman, Ron Raab and Dr Jorgen Vesti-Neilsen has been invaluable in keeping me up to date with the research in the low carb/diabetes community over the last ten years. This has been very necessary when there has been such a concerted effort to avoid changing the status quo in the UK.

I have made many internet friends of other parents of diabetic children and adult diabetics who have given much helpful advice on how to cope with the condition and often have just been there to listen. Janet in particular has helped expand my repertoire in the kitchen.

Emma would like to thank her mum and dad, Jock and Brenda, who made a huge effort to treat her like a normal child and teenager whilst growing up. She thanks them, and her sisters, for their patience when diabetes-related grumpiness took its toll. Thanks to Sandy and his voyage of discovery about what it's like to live with a diabetic, and thanks too to Heather Maxwell for teaching me much, much more about diabetes.

We'd both like to say particular thanks to those who submitted their low carb stories for the testimonial section, and we wish you all continued good health. Grateful thanks too, to Michelle Kay for her help in transferring the first edition of this book to Kindle format.

We've found the experience of co-writing informative, educational and interesting – a book such as this needs different skills, and we've both (hopefully!) complemented each other in the process of writing.

APPENDIX A

WARM UP AND MORE STRETCHES

When you embark on our suggested strength training programmes – either the body weight or weights exercises, we suggest you start with a light warm-up programme.

We've also included some further stretches you can incorporate into the routine we proposed in Chapter 6. You can do stretches every day – and this is recommended for maximum flexibility and to ensure you are still capable of cutting your own toenails in your old age – but you should not stretch cold muscles so do this after either exercise or having done the warm-up first. Many people skip the stretches at the end of a workout, but they are important.

Warm up Exercises

To warm up, start by marching on the spot. Start slowly for one minute or so and then build up the momentum by making your arms work harder and lifting your knees up higher. Do this for about two minutes.

Do arm circles forward for 30 seconds and backwards for 30 seconds.

Do jumping jacks for 30 seconds and then circle your head eight times to the left and then eight times to the right.

Circle your hips eight times to the left and eight times to the right.

Finish by jogging on the spot or 30 seconds and 30-seconds-worth of jumping jacks.

More Stretches

Cross over stretch – lie on your back, bring one knee to your chest and extend the other leg. Bring your bent knee over your body, so it faces one way and your head the other.

Hamstring stretch – lie on your back. Extend both legs. Now bring one leg up to 90 degrees till you feel a pull on the back of your leg. Hold.

Pyriformis stretch – lie on your back and bend both knees. Bring one leg up and cross the ankle of that leg over the knee of the leg on the floor. Put your hands behind the knee resting on the floor and bring it towards your face until you feel a stretch in the buttock of the leg that is crossed over your knee.

Pretzel – sit up with your legs extended in front of you. Cross one leg over the other. Turn your torso towards the extended leg and grip your bent thigh with the arm of your extended leg. Turn your head and press the leg till you feel the stretch in your spine.

Mermaid – sit on the floor with both legs tucked in at one side. Lean over those legs with your torso with one arm extended over your head. Hold onto your foot on the floor with the other hand (to stop you from toppling over). Hold the stretch feeling it down one side of the torso. Repeat on the other side.

Cross legs side bend – standing up cross your legs in front of you at the ankle. Put one arm on your waist and extend the other over your head. Bend to the side supporting your waist. Repeat on the other side.

Cross legs forward bend – NB do not do this stretch if you have proliferative retinopathy. Standing up in the same cross legged position, bend forward over your legs. This gives a good stretch along the back of the leg and is relaxing for your neck and shoulders. Repeat on the other side.

Shoulder circle – standing up rotate your arms in wide circles in both directions.

Cross-legged forward bends – sit cross-legged. Bend your torso forward over your knees till you feel a stretch in the buttocks. Do the same with the other leg in front.

One leg kneel – kneel with your upper legs and torso vertical. Put one leg out in front and place your hand on that knee. Press your buttock down with the other leg till you feel a stretch in the front of the thigh. Repeat with the other leg.

Runners stretch – extend one leg out and the other behind. Place your hands in front of you and bend the front of your body over the front leg. Press into the heel of your back leg. Feel the stretch along both legs and the heel. Repeat on both sides.

APPENDIX B

STRENGTH TRAINING WITH WEIGHTS

Once you have built up your strength using our body weight exercises, move on using weights.

You will need a set of dumbbells. You can buy adjustable dumbbells. The weights increase by 2.5 kg increments. These are expensive, but it means that you don't end up with lots of different weights hidden behind your couch.

Single weight dumbbells, on the other hand, can be bought in 0.5 and 1kg increments which are better for beginners. Men can use 5 pounds (2.5kg) as light weights and 10 pounds (4-5kg) as heavy weights. Women can use 5 pounds (2.5kg) as heavy weights and 3 pounds (1.5kg) as light weights. These will be reasonable starting weights if you are not used to weight training. You can build up weights and numbers of sets gradually as your fitness level improves.

[There is an old-fashioned and incorrect view that using weights will bulk you up if you are a woman, which is simply not true. Female body builders lift hefty weights, eat a very, very high protein, low fat and low-carb diet and work out for hours a day to achieve their physique. A half-hour/40-minute routine followed two or three times a week with moderate or even heavy weights will tone you up, but will not add bulk.]

This routine uses dumbbells and alternates upper and lower body exercises to get your heart rate up. Take 30 seconds to one-minute rest between the sets of exercise for the same body part. If you alternate the sets between two different muscle groups, e.g. 8 reps upper body and then 8 reps lower body, you don't usually need recovery time between exercises.

A basic method of weight training is 6-8 reps for men and 8-10 reps for women. Once you can do the top rep count comfortably, you need to up the weight for that exercise. You may only manage the first set with the higher weight to start with. That's fine. Do all reps slowly to minimise the effects of momentum (which otherwise helps you cheat!).

If you are starting out at 10 minutes a day, just go through as many exercises as you can in that time and pick up where you left off on the next strength day.

Arnold press: hold the dumbbells in front of your chest with your palms facing you. Raise the weights above your head and as you do rotate the weights, so your thumbs face each other. Use light weights then as you improve go onto heavy weights.

Squat: hold the weights with your palms facing your legs. Stick your bottom out and lower it as if you are going to sit on a chair. When your legs are at right angles, 90 degrees to each other stand up slowly and squeeze your buttock muscles as you do. Use heavy weights.

Row: hold the weights out in front of you, palms facing each other at waist height. Bend your knees slightly. Bring them in towards you and behind you. Bring your shoulder blades together as you pull them behind you. Return the weights to the starting position and do it again. Use heavy weights.

Stationary lunge each side: stand with your feet just over hip width apart. Hold the weights in both hands at your sides palms facing each other. Take a step back with one leg. Keep your torso upright. Bend your legs and bring your bottom down until your knees are at 90 degrees. Squeeze your legs as you come back up. Use heavy weights.

Lateral raise: stand upright. Bring the weights palms facing each other in front of you at groin level. Raise them up to shoulder level but don't go higher than this. Hold for a few seconds at shoulder level then lower slowly. Use light weights.

Deadlifts: stand upright with the weights held palms against your thighs. Bend forward from the hips as far as you can, keeping the weights close to your legs. Straighten up slowly. Use heavy weights. If you are quite stiff, you may bend your knees a bit. Men are usually a lot stiffer than women on this exercise.

Front raise: stand upright. Hold the weights as if you have jugs of water in your hands. Bring the arms up to shoulder level but not further. Use light weights.

Leg press: stand in the same position as for the stationary lunge, BUT bend at the waist so that your head is nearer your front foot. From this position, put your heavy weights on the floor either side of one foot. Lift them up to your knee level with your palms facing each other. Lower them again.

Shoulder raise: stand upright. Hold the weights palms towards your body. Now lift both of them up in the midline as if you are zipping up a coat. Bring your weights to just under your chin then lower and repeat. Use heavy weights.

Sumo squat: stand with your legs wide apart. Put the heavy weights on your thighs at mid-thigh level holding on with the palm facing the thigh. Bend down like a ballerina and then stand up squeezing your thighs and buttocks.

Hammer biceps curl: hold the heavy weights like jugs of water with your arms close to your sides. Bring your arm up like you are going to drink but keep your head up. Put it down. This exercise strengthens the forearm as well as the biceps.

Calf raises: hold onto the back of a chair. Raise up on both calves and slowly go down. When you can do this easily stand on a telephone book (for example) with the spine towards you to increase the range of movement. You can also do this one leg at a time with the other leg tucked behind the heel of the other for a greater weight load.

Push-ups: start doing these on your knees with your forearms out in front of you and your arms wider than your chest. Go up and down slowly. Once you can do 3 sets of 8 increase the challenge by doing press ups on your toes.

Bottom/hamstring squeezes: lie on your back arms by your sides. Place your knees on the floor away from your bottom hip width apart. Raise your bottom off the floor and squeeze your buttocks and hamstrings. You can make this harder by putting one leg over the other thigh to give extra weight or holding one leg at the level of the knee of the moving leg.

Triceps French press: lie on the ground with light weights in each hand. Bend the elbow to a right angle and slowly bring the weights towards each ear.

Plank: kneel on the floor. Put both hands out in front of you at shoulder level and push up to your knees. Hold this for 20 seconds and build up gradually to one minute. When you can do this go up to your toes and build that up too. This exercise strengthens the wrists which are a common fracture site. If your wrists bother you put your forearms on the floor instead.

Standing weight turns: Hold two weights out in front of you with your elbows bent at waist height. Keep your head and hips facing forward but bring the weights to one side and then the other at waist height. Pretend there is a wall behind you and stop before the weights go behind you. This strengthens your oblique abdominal muscles.

APPENDIX C

EXTRA SAMPLE MENUS

W e've added in another week of a sample menu plan for you. This is quite a low carbohydrate plan. You can mix and match the meals to suit, so long as you take account of the carbohydrate totals for each meal and the total carbohydrates for your overall day.

DAY 1

Breakfast: 1 slice almond bread, sugar reduced marmalade, 2 boiled eggs

10g carbs

Lunch: Meat stew and one orange

15g carbs

Dinner: roast lamb, cheese, one apple, 20g plain chocolate (70% cocoa solids)

25g carbs

TOTAL CARBS – 50g

DAY 2

Breakfast: 3 low carb pancakes, butter, 2 boiled eggs

10g carbs

Lunch: Smoked salmon, 3 scrambled eggs/butter, 2 large chopped tomatoes

10g carbs

Dinner: roast duck, home-made raspberry sauce, 2 small roast potatoes, 150g mushrooms

30g carbs

Snack: cheese, 50g peanuts

5g carbs

TOTAL CARBS – 55g

DAY 3

Breakfast: 2 soft-boiled eggs, 100g asparagus spears

3g carbs

Lunch: lentil soup, Asian spiced chicken and steamed cabbage

30g carbs

Dinner: prawns with garlic mayonnaise, 100g salad leaves and cheese

5g carbs

TOTAL CARBS – 38g

DAY 4

Breakfast: Three scrambled eggs with 50g chopped smoked salmon, three medium sliced tomatoes and one orange

20g carbs

Lunch: roast chicken and a big salad with olive oil/white wine vinegar dressing

10g carbs

Dinner: crab and mayonnaise, chopped spring onions, cheese and one apple

15g carbs

TOTAL CARBS – 45g

DAY 5

Breakfast: 2 rashers bacon, two fried eggs and one slice black pudding with two medium chopped tomatoes

17g carbs

Lunch: 6 scallops, 6 king prawns with butter, one sliced chilli and spring onions, one apple

20g carbs

Dinner: roast chicken, garlic mayonnaise, large salad and one slice low-carb Victoria Sponge

20g carbs

TOTAL CARBS: 57g

DAY 6

Breakfast: omelette made with 2 eggs, chilli and cheese, one apple

15g carbs

Lunch: Beef stew with carrot and peas

20g carbs

Dinner: baked salmon with steamed broccoli, low-carb chocolate coconut custard

15g carbs

1 glass red wine, 50g peanuts

TOTAL CARBS: 55g

DAY 7

Breakfast: Turkey rashers with 100g fried mushrooms, one orange

15g carbs

Lunch: 3 slices roast beef/horseradish, one pear and cheese

15g carbs

Dinner: Mozzarella cheese, tomato and basil salad; moussaka; raspberries and double cream

One glass red wine

25g carbs

TOTAL CARBS – 55g

APPENDIX D

ADAPTING FAVOURITE RECIPES TO SUIT YOUR NEW DIET

If you already own a lot of recipe books, you may be looking at them in despair, wondering if they are now obsolete and ought to be donated to your local charity shop...

Alternatively, you may be like the majority of the population – owner of a lot of cookery books of which only a handful of recipes have ever been attempted.

Anyway, many recipe books will have plenty of recipes which can fit perfectly into your new low carb way of eating. Look out for fish, meat and egg recipes which focus mainly on protein and vegetables and do not use rice, pasta, potatoes and flour – although the odd spoonful of flour is not an issue.

You can use chopped nuts instead of bread crumbs as a topping for fish or chicken, and you can use ground almonds as a thickener for sauces in place of flour. Double cream can also thicken up sauces, as can egg yolks and guar gum (add this slowly to prevent clumping).

Cauliflower can be used in place of mashed potatoes (cook and purée with a little butter).

A meat thermometer is a beneficial device which when used correctly virtually guarantees that the meat will be cooked to your satisfaction. You will probably be roasting more meat and poultry than usual because the left overs can be used for more than one meal. Given the expense of meat you really want it to turn out well.

There are many different low carb recipe books that cater for the low carb baker. Sponge cakes and pancakes made from ground almonds taste better than the flour equivalent, but the consistency is always denser. To achieve some lift to the product you often need to beat the egg whites separately and fold in using a large metal spoon at the end, just before it gets cooked or baked. When you add baking powder or other raising agents you have only 25 minutes to get it in the oven before the results will be impaired. For even baking of a cake or bread, mix the dry ingredients together first so they are evening blended and then add gradually to the mixed wet ingredients.

For sugar substitutes, you have a wide choice. Stevia powder or liquid is a very useful substance which has little or no caloric value. It is good to add to fruit dishes or cheesecakes. Where it falls down is in some of the low carb baking where the sugar is performing a bulking action such as in sponge cakes or muffins. Here you would probably use a granular sugar substitute such as Splenda, erythritol or xylitol.

None of the sugar substitutes gives the caramelisation effect of real sugar so you may need to use the occasional teaspoonful on the top of pies or custards when necessary.

APPENDIX E

CARB FACTORS

The carb factor is the percentage of foods which is carbohydrate. It is a particularly useful measurement for working out the carbohydrate value of fresh food and vegetables, as these items tend not to be a standard size. If you know the carb factor of an apple, for instance (13% of an apple is carbohydrate), you can then work out how many carbs your apple has, no matter its size. To access the full listings, visit http://www.carbfactors.com/

This table is from the UDSA site:

BREADS & GRAINS

Bagel 0.56

Biscuits 0.45

Bread 0.53

Macaroni, plain 0.23

Muffins 0.45

Pancakes, prepared 0.44

Rice, cooked 0.24

Spaghetti, plain 0.28

CEREALS, COLD

Cheerios 0.70

Corn Flakes 0.84

Grapenuts 0.83

Puffed Wheat 0.77

Rice Krispies 0.88

Total 0.79

Wheaties 0.80

CEREALS, HOT

Cream of Wheat 0.14

Oatmeal 0.10

Roman Meal 0.14

COMBINATION FOODS

Lasagne 0.16

Macaroni & Cheese 0.20

Pizza 0.28

DESSERTS & CANDIES

Angel Food Cake 0.60

Banana Bread 0.46

Brownie with nuts 0.50

Cookies

1. Animal 0.80

2. Chocolate Chip 0.59

3. Oatmeal Raisin 0.72

Doughnut, cake 0.52

Fudge with nuts 0.69

Peanut Brittle 0.73

Pies

1. Apple 0.37
2. Lemon Meringue 0.38
3. Pecan 0.23
4. Pumpkin 0.23

FRUITS

Apple 0.13

Apricots

1. fresh 0.13
2. dried 0.60

Banana 0.20

Cantaloupe 0.08

Grapes 0.14

Peaches, fresh 0.10

Pears, fresh 0.15

Prunes, dried 0.67

Strawberries 0.08

Watermelon 0.06

SNACKS

Almonds 0.19

Cashews 0.26

Corn chips 0.57

Crackers

Graham 0.73

Saltine 0.70

Marshmallows 0.78

Peanut butter 0.17

Popcorn, no butter 0.78

Potato chips 0.50

Walnuts 0.15

VEGETABLES

Avocado 0.05

Beans

1. Green, raw 0.07
2. Green, cooked 0.05

Kidney, lima, pinto, red 0.21

Beets, boiled 0.07

Carrots

Raw 0.10

Cooked 0.07

Corn

1. Steamed 0.19
2. Creamed 0.20

Potatoes

1. Baked 0.21
2. Boiled 0.15
3. French Fries 0.34

Squash

1. Summer, cooked 0.03
2. Winter, baked 0.15
3. Winter, boiled 0.09

APPENDIX F

HBA1C CONVERSIONS

Since June 2011, the way HbA1C values are presented has changed and they are now reported in a mmol/mol format instead of a percentage. It can be quite challenging moving from one measurement to the other and making sense of it, so here is a list of measurements and their conversions.

HbA1c Percentage/mmol/mol

5.0	31
5.1	32
5.2	33
5.3	34
5.4	36
5.5	37
5.6	38
5.7	39
5.8	40
5.9	41
6.0	42
6.1	43
6.2	44
6.3	45

6.4	46
6.5	48
6.6	49
6.7	50
6.8	51
6.9	52
7.0	53
7.1	54
7.2	55
7.3	56
7.4	57
7.5	58
7.6	60
7.7	61
7.8	62
7.9	63
8.0	64
8.1	65
8.2	66
8.3	67
8.4	68
8.5	69
8.6	70
8.7	72
8.8	73
8.9	74
9.0	75
9.1	76
9.2	77
9.3	78
9.4	79
9.5	80

9.6	81
9.7	83
9.8	84
9.9	85
10.0	86
10.1	87
10.2	88
10.3	89
10.4	90
10.5	91
10.6	92
10.7	93
10.8	95
10.9	96
11.0	97
11.1	98
11.2	99
11.3	100
11.4	101
11.5	102
11.6	103
11.7	104
11.8	105
11.9	107
12.0	108
12.1	109
12.2	110
12.3	111
12.4	112
12.5	113
12.6	114
12.7	115

12.8	118
12.9	117
13.0	119

APPENDIX G

USEFUL FORMS

B lood Glucose Monitoring Sheet or records give you a format you can use to record your own blood sugar levels.

You can download samples here - https://www.diabetesnet.com/pdfs/smart_chart.pdf

There are also apps you can use to record your blood sugar levels, such as mysugr, Diabetes Pal and Dbees.

Here is an explanation of useful apps (and mostly free) apps you can use: http://www.diabeticconnect.com/diabetes-information-articles/general/1935-diabetes-apps-the-best-blood-sugar-and-medicine-management-apps

We have also included a diabetes concerns form, which you can fill in before visiting your own GP or diabetic clinic to ensure that your worries and concerns are addressed. (Thanks to Martha Funnell)

DIABETES CONCERNS ASSESSMENT FORM		
Patient Name:		
Date of Birth:		
Please answer the following questions before your visit. Your answers will help ensure that your concerns are addressed.		
1	What is hardest or causing you most concern about caring for your diabetes at this time? (e.g. following a diet/medication/stress)	
2	Please write down a few words about what you find difficult or frustrating about the concern you mentioned above.	
3	How would you describe your thoughts or feelings about this issue? (e.g. confused/angry/curious/ worried/frustrated/depressed/hopeful)	
4	What would you like us to do during your visit to help address your concern? (please circle A, B, and/or C – all that apply to you)	
	A	*Work with me to come up with a plan to address this issue.*
	B	*I don't expect a solution, I just want you to understand what it is like for me.*
	C	*Refer me to another health professional or other community services.*
5	I would like answers to the following questions at this visit:	
6	I would like answers to the following questions at some future visit:	
7	Other: (please explain)	
8	Action taken by GP/Nurse:	
FOR ADMIN USE ONLY		

Name: _____

Age: _____

CHI no: _____

Date of birth: _____

Address: _____

Phone numbers: _____

Reason for admission: _____

Consultant: _____

GP: _____

Relevant medical history for subject of admission: _____

_____

Diabetes history: _____

Type: _____

What age diagnosed: _____

Any complications: _____

_____

Last HbAIC: _____

Diabetes consultant: _____

Hospitals currently attended: _____

Past medical history for other conditions: _____

_____

Operations: _____

_____

Serious illnesses: _____

_____

Trauma: _____

Blood transfusions: _____

Fits/Infections/Head injuries: _____

_____

Menarche/contraception/pregnancies/menopause: _____

_____

Dental:_____

_____

Eyesight: _____

Retinopathy: _____

_____

Condition of feet:_____

Proteinuria: _____

_____

BP:_____

Drugs: _____

INSULIN: detailed information types, doses, meal adjustments

_____

Non- prescription medication: _____

Allergies: _____

_____

Smokes/Drinks/ other substances: _____

Mental health: _____

Dr. Katharine Morrison and Emma Baird

Other: _____

_____

Height: _____

Weight: _____

BMI: _____

Dietary preferences: _____

_____

Usual exercise routine/ mobility issues:_____

_____

Social: _____

Type of house: _____

Access eg keypad, stairs, bath, shower: _____

Who lives with you: _____

Helpers: _____

Aids in the house: _____

Occupation: _____

Driving: _____

Hobbies/sports: _____

APPENDIX H

HOW TO IMPROVE LOW SELF-ESTEEM

The path to being fit and slim takes a multitude of very small steps. We are products of our genetics and daily habits. Make small progressive changes to those daily habits, and over time you will see beneficial change.

Think about the body, health, self-control and confidence that you want to achieve. How does a person who is like this organise their day? How do they eat? What? When? How do they look after their emotional health? Take time to think about how a person like this lives (study them covertly if necessary). Now, incorporate one or two of their useful and healthful daily habits into your own day.

It can be helpful to start the day by doing something for yourself. This can be as simple as putting on a lovely perfume, putting on make-up or your favourite colour of top, or taking your dog a brief walk to the paper shop and having a chat with other customers.

Look on exercise as "me" time and enjoy the moment and the rewards. Try to spend some time every day outdoors enjoying nature. Bring some of nature indoors, for example, flowers or a plant to brighten up your life.

At the end of the day, it is helpful to spend half an hour before you go to bed winding down. Have a warm bath, listen to soothing music, or read a non-demanding book. TV or being on a computer close to bedtime isn't helpful as it can interfere with your sleep.

We all have emotional needs, and sometimes they are just not met. Over-eating can provide a (very) temporary emotional lift. The requirements as stated by Human Givens are:

1. A sense of security in all major areas of your life

2. Feeling that you receive enough attention

3. Able to give others enough attention

4. Feeling in control of your life most of the time

5. Feeling connected to some part of the wider community

6. Able to obtain privacy when you need it

7. Have an intimate relationship with another person (one where you are physically and emotionally accepted for who you are by at least one other person or animal)

8. A feeling of being emotionally connected to others

9. A feeling that you have a status that is acknowledged

10. Feeling competent and achieving things in at least one area of your life

11. Being mentally and/or physically stretched in ways that give you a sense that life is meaningful.

Are your needs being met?

When you realise the areas of your life that need to change, you can explore how to do this with help from your friends, self-help books, or referral to a counsellor or therapist.

Have you got a serious eating disorder?

If you eat to excess and then vomit it up or starve yourself afterwards to compensate, then this is a problem called bulimia. Referral to an eating disorders clinic may help. It is worth dealing with this because binge eating is bad for your blood sugar control, and the vomiting is bad for your teeth and blood salts control. The root of it is usually low self-esteem. What starts out as an apparently harmless habit makes you feel even worse about yourself.

The website "Diabetics with Eating Disorders" http://dwed.org.uk/ can help if you are a type one diabetic who is manipulating insulin to lose weight, anorexic, or engages in binging and/or vomiting.

ENDNOTES

[1] Dr Bernstein's Diabetes Solution by Dr Richard K. Bernstein (Brown and Little)

[2] Diabet Med. 2014 Feb;31(2):227-31. doi: 10.1111/dme.12305. Epub 2013 Sep 19.Medical and psychological outcomes for young adults with Type 1 diabetes: no improvement despite recent advances in diabetes care. Johnson B1, Elliott J, Scott A, Heller S, Eiser C.

[3] Diabetes UK - http://www.diabetes.org.uk/About_us/What-we-say/Statistics/Diabetes-prevalence-2013/

[4] American Diabetes Association - http://professional.diabetes.org/admin/UserFiles/0%20-%20Sean/FastFacts%20March%202013.pdf

[5] Antonio Ceriello MD, Point: Post prandial glucose levels are a clinically important treatment target. Diabetes Care. Aug 2010; 33(8): 1905–1907.

[6] National Institutes of Health: http://www.nlm.nih.gov/medlineplus/magazine/issues/summer08/articles/summer08pg14-15.html

[7] Bernstein R K. Virtually continuous euglycemia for 5 yr in a labile juvenile-onset diabetic patient under noninvasive closed-loop control. *Diabetes Care* 1980;3:140-143

[8] Diabetology & Metabolic Syndrome - http://www.dmsjournal.com/content/4/1/23

[9] Am J Med. 1987 Feb;82(2):213-20. **Deleterious metabolic effects of high-carbohydrate, sucrose-containing diets in patients with non-insulin-dependent diabetes mellitus.** Coulston AM, Hollenbeck CB, Swislocki AL, Chen YD, Reaven GM.

10a R. Feinman et al: Dietary carbohydrate restriction as the first approach in diabetes management. Critical review and evidence base. Nutrition July14 DOI:10.1016/j.nut.2014.06.011

[10] Healthcare Improvement Scotland - http://www.sign.ac.uk/guidelines/fulltext/116/

[11] Byron J. Richards CCN Mastering Leptin Wellness Resources Books

[12] Accurso et al Dietary carbohydrate restriction in type 2 diabetes mellitus and metabolic syndrome: time for a critical appraisal Nutrition and Metabolism April 2008

13a R Feinman et al: Dietary carbohydrate restriction as the first approach in diabetes management. Critical review and evidence base. Nutrition July 14. DOI:10.1016/j.nut.2014.06.011.

[13] People who type 1 diabetes often develop coeliac disease and vice versa. Both are autoimmune conditions. https://www.coeliac.org.uk/coeliac-disease/associated-conditions-and-complications/type-1-diabetes/

[14] http://www.health.harvard.edu/newsweek/Glycemic_index_and_glycemic_load_for_100_foods.htm

[15] *Mastering Leptin: Your Guide to Permanent Weight Loss and Optimum Health*

[16] The DCCT was funded by the US National Institute of Diabetes and Digestive and Kidney Diseases between 1983 and 1993. It proved that keeping blood sugar levels as close to normal as possible slows the onset and progression of the eye, kidney and nerve damage caused by diabetes. In fact, the trial demonstrated that any sustained lowering of blood sugars helps, even if the person has a history of poor control.

[17] Ouyang X. Fructose consumption as a risk factor for non-alcoholic fatty liver disease, Journal of Hepatology Volume 48, Issue 6, June 2008, Pages 993–999

[18] Day CP, Review Non-alcoholic fatty liver disease: The mist gradually clears, Journal of Hepatology Volume 48, Supplement 1, 2008, Pages S104–S112

[19] Naniwadekar A. Nutritional Recommendations for Patients with Non-Alcoholic Fatty Liver Disease: An Evidence Based Review. Practical Gastroenterology Feb 2010.

[20] Dr Bernstein's Diabetes Solution

[21] Dr Bernstein's Diabetes Solution

[22] Waldron S: **Controversies in the dietary management of diabetes in childhood and adolescence**. *Br J Hosp Med* 1996, 56(8):450-454

[23] Heinemann L: **Variability of insulin absorption and insulin action**.

[24] Dr Bernstein's Diabetes Solution

[25] Hypoglycemia in the Diabetes Control and Complications Trial The Diabetes Control and Complications Trial Research Group Diabetes February 1997 vol. 46 no. 2 271-286

[26] Wiegand S et al Clinical Study: Daily insulin requirement of children and adolescents with type one diabetes: effect of age, gender, body mass index and mode of therapy. European Journal of Endocrinology (2008) 158 543-549.

[27] Gleason C E, Gonzalez, M et al. Determinants of glucose toxicity and its reversibility in the pancreatic islet -cell line, HIT-T15. *Am J Physiol Endocrinol Metab* 2000;279:E997-E1002

[28] Garber A.J. Incretin Effects on -Cell Function, Replication, and Mass The human perspective Diabetes Care May 2011 vol. 34 no. Supplement 2 S258-S263

[29] See Vicky's story in the Success Stories chapter.

[30] Valko M. Free radicals, metals and antioxidants in oxidative stress-induced cancer Chemico-Biological Interactions. Volume 160, Issue 1, 10 March 2006, Pages 1–40

[31] Yam D, Eliraz A, Berry EM Department of Membrane Research and Biophysics, Weizmann Institute of Science, Rehovot, Israel. Israel Journal of Medical Sciences [1996, 32(11):1134-1143] Diet and disease--the Israeli paradox: possible dangers of a high omega-6 polyunsaturated fatty acid diet.

[32] http://www.cancer.gov/cancertopics/factsheet/Risk/obesity National Cancer Institute USA

[33] http://www.aicr.org/continuous-update-project/reports/ovarian-cancer-2014-report.pdf

[34] Dreon D M, Fernstrom H A et al. Low-density lipoprotein subclass patterns and lipoprotein response to a reduced-fat diet in men. *FASEB J* 1994;8:121-126

[35] Krauss R M. Dietary and genetic probes of atherogenic dyslipidemia. *Arterioscler Thromb Vasc Biol* 2005;25:2265-2272

[36] Evidence for an Independent and Cumulative Effect of Postprandial Hypertriglyceridemia and Hyperglycemia on Endothelial Dysfunction and Oxidative Stress Generation Effects of Short- and Long-Term Simvastatin Treatment

Antonio Ceriello, MD; et al Circulation.2002; 106: 1211-1218 Published online before print August 19, 2002

[37] http://www.oxidativestressresource.org/

[38] Proceedings of the Nutrition Society Volume 60 / Issue 03 / August 2001, pp 349-356 Symposium on 'New perspectives on adipose tissue function' Pro-inflammatory cytokines and adipose tissue Simon W. Coppacka1

[39] Circulation.2007;   115:   450-458   December   26,   2006 Triglycerides   and   the   Risk   of   Coronary   Heart   Disease 10 158 Incident Cases Among 262 525 Participants in 29 Western Prospective Studies Nadeem Sarwar

[40] Volek J S, Feinman R D. Carbohydrate restriction improves the features of metabolic syndrome. Metabolic syndrome may be defined by the response to carbohydrate restriction. *Nutr Metab (Lond)* 2005;2:31

[41] Assmann G, Schulte H, von Eckardstein A, Huang Y. High-density lipoprotein cholesterol as a predictor of coronary heart disease risk. The PROCAM experience and pathophysiological implications for reverse cholesterol transport. Atherosclerosis 1996;124(suppl):S11–20.

[42] Mensink RP, Zock PL, Kester AD, Katan MB. Effects of dietary fatty acids and carbohydrates on the ratio of serum total to HDL cholesterol and on serum lipids and apolipoproteins: a meta-analysis of 60 controlled trials. Am J Clin Nutr 2003;77:1146–55.

[43] Comparison of Effects of High and Low Carbohydrate Diets on Plasma Lipoproteins and Insulin Sensitivity in Patients With Mild NIDDM Abhimanyu Garg, Scott M Grundy and Roger H Unger Diabetes October 1992 vol. 41 no. 10 1278-1285

[44] The American Journal of Cardiology Volume 96, Issue 3, 1 August 2005, Pages 399–404 Is There a Simple Way to Identify Insulin-Resistant Individuals at Increased Risk of Cardiovascular Disease? Tracey McLaughlin et al.

272

[45] JAMA. 2006 Feb 8;295(6):655-66.Low-fat dietary pattern and risk of cardiovascular disease: the Women's Health Initiative Randomized Controlled Dietary Modification Trial. Howard BV1,et al

[46] AMA. 1982 Sep 24;248(12):1465-77. Multiple risk factor intervention trial. Risk factor changes and mortality results. Multiple Risk Factor Intervention Trial Research Group.

[47] TD Noakes Critique: The women's health initiative randomised controlled dietary modification trial: an inconvenient finding and the diet-heart hypothesis. Nov 2013 Vol 103 No 11 SAMJ

[48] WB Kannel T Gordon The Framingham Dietary Study: diet and the regulation of serum cholesterol (Sect 24) Washington DC, Department of Health Education and Welfare 1970.

[49] Barter P J, Ballantyne C M et al. Apo B versus cholesterol in estimating cardiovascular risk and in guiding therapy; report of the thirty–person/ten-country panel. *J Intern Med* 2006:259:247-258

[50] Kristin Castorini and Lois Jovanovic Pregnancy and Diabetes Management Clinical Chemistry **February 2011 vol. 57 no. 2 221-230**

[51] Major C A, Henry M J et al. The effects of carbohydrate restriction in patients with diet-controlled gestational diabetes. *Obstet Gynecol* 1998;91:600-604

[52] Diabetes Self-Management, Strike the Spike New and Improved 2010, Gary Scheiner MS, CDE – Integrated Diabetes Services LLC

[53] EDITORIAL Intensive Glycemic Control in the ACCORD and ADVANCE Trials

Robert G. Dluhy, M.D., and Graham T. McMahon, M.D., M.M.Sc.

N Engl J Med 2008; 358:2630-2633June 12, 2008DOI: 10.1056/ NEJMe0804182

[54] Diabetes UK: (http://www.diabetes.org.uk/Guide-to-diabetes/Recipes/)

[55] American Diabetes Association (http://www.diabetes.org/food-and-fitness/food/ what-can-i-eat/making-healthy-food-choices.html)

[56] Based on small servings of 30g cereal, 150ml milk, a small roll, tomato and lentil soup, 100g potatoes, 75g fruit salad packed in juice and three small bran crackers.

[57] Dr Bernstein's Diabetes Solution. "The law of small numbers". NB Dr Bernstein has had type one diabetes since the age of 12. He was a successful engineer before he retrained as a physician at the age of 45. He had applied engineering principles to achieving normal blood sugars, but to his dismay found the medical profession were not interested. He thought that if he became a doctor he would have greater influence on changing the prognosis for diabetics for the better. He has had a long and hard struggle, but science has always been on his side. He is now in his 80s, still works full time as a diabetic physician, and has reversed almost all of the complications he had from his diabetes and has truly been a pioneer in normal blood sugars for diabetics. Maybe the tipping point has come?

[58] Nielsen J V, Jönsson E, Ivarsson A. A low carbohydrate diet in type 1 diabetes: clinical experience - a brief report. Ups J Med Sci 2005;110:267-273.

[59] Nielsen JV, Gando C, Joensson E, Paulsson C. Low carbohydrate diet in type 1 diabetes, long term improvement and adherence: A clinical audit. Diabetology & Metabolic Syndrome 2012, 4:23 doi:10.1186/1758-5996-4-23

[60] Bernstein R K. Virtually continuous euglycemia for 5 yr in a labile juvenile-onset diabetic patient under non-invasive closed-loop control. Diabetes Care 1980;3:140-143

[61] Dietary ketosis is a normal phenomenon that occurs when there is a relative lack in dietary carbohydrate. The body uses up body fat for fuel and a side effect is the spilling of ketones, a by product of fat metabolism, into the blood stream, breath and urine. The amounts are small and not dangerous.

[62] Ketoacidosis or DKA is a potentially life-threatening condition which occurs when a severe or relative lack of insulin causes the liver to break down other body tissues in high amounts and is most common in people with type 1 diabetes. Left untreated, DKA can be fatal.

[63] The standard recommendation for carbohydrates in the diet are 55-60%. 20% of carbs in a 2,500 calorie diet is roughly 500 calories.

[64] http://www.qualityhealth.com/news/low-carb-diets-work-overweight-diabetics-8989

[65] **Low glycaemic index or low glycaemic load diets for overweight and obesity** DE Thomas, EJ Elliott, L Baur *Cochrane Database of Systematic Reviews* 2008 Issue 1

[66] Dr Bernstein's Diabetes Solution.

[67] British National Formulary BNF 66 Sept 13-March 14 also at bnf.org

[68] Think Like a Pancreas By Gary Scheiner MS CDE Marlowe and Company

[69] Dr Bernstein's Diabetes Solution

[70] Dr Bernstein's Diabetes Solution

[71] Dr Bernstein's Diabetes Solution

[72] Gannon MC, Nuttall FQ. Effect of a high-protein, low carbohydrate diet on blood glucose control in people with type two diabetes. Diabetes. 2004;53:2375-2382.

[73] BNF 66

[74] http://www.diabetes.org.uk/Documents/Professionals/News,%20updates,%20prizes%20and%20alerts/Driving-diabetes-professional-guidance0212.pdf

[75] Metabolic syndrome is not an illness itself, but it refers to risk factors such as high blood pressure, high blood sugar levels, unhealthy cholesterol levels and high amounts of belly fat. Such risk factors make heart disease more likely.

[76] Nielsen JV, Joensson E. Low-carbohydrate diet in type two diabetes: stable improvement of bodyweight and glycemic control during 44 months follow up. *Nutrition & Metabolism* 2008, 5:1. Nielsen JV, Gando C, Joensson E, Paulsson C. Low carbohydrate diet in type 1 diabetes, long term improvement and adherence: A clinical audit. *Diabetology & Metabolic Syndrome* 2012, 4:23

[77] **Pregnancy and Diabetes Management: Advances and Controversies Kristin Castorino[1] and Lois Jovanovic[1],*** Clinical Chemistry**February 2011 vol. 57 no. 2 221-230**

[78] Think Like a Pancreas. Page 53 table 4.2 Gary Scheiner Marlowe and Company

[79] Ref: Wei N, Zheng H, Nathan D: Empirically establishing blood glucose targets to achieve HbA1C goals. Diabetes Care Feb 10 2014.

[80] Pumping Insulin by John Walsh and Ruth Roberts (Chapter 18 is devoted to pregnancy). ISBN-13: 978-1884804861

[81] Schwartz F and Marling C. Use of Automated Bolus Calculators for Diabetes Management. US Endocrinology. 2013;124-127.

[82] Net carbs are the carbohydrates in foods after the amount of fibre has been subtracted because fibre content does not affect your blood sugar levels.

[83] Rassam A G, Zeise T M et al. Optimal administration of lispro insulin in hyperglyemic type 1 diabetes. *Diabetes Care* 1999;22:133-136

[84] It is sometimes easier to stick to a low-carbohydrate plan when you are eating out if you order two starters, rather than a starter or a main meal or just a main meal.

[85] Medline Plus report on chromium - http://www.nlm.nih.gov/medlineplus/druginfo/natural/932.html

[86] Dr Bernstein's Diabetes Solution has thorough, sensible and effective information on these subjects. The key is early recognition and knowing exactly what to do and what the limits of home treatment are before a crisis develops. Keeping a copy of the book at home and away would be prudent.

[87] Interview with Jimmy Moore on the Livin La Vida Low Carb show 2012

[88] Lipids October 2010, Volume 45, Issue 10, pp 947-962, Limited Effect of Dietary Saturated Fat on Plasma Saturated Fat in the Context of a Low Carbohydrate Diet Cassandra E. Forsythe et al.

[89] Jacqui Troughton Practical Diabetes International 2003

[90] The State of the Nation by Diabetes UK in 2013 reports that 80% of expenditure for diabetes is on the COMPLICATIONS and only 20% is for the management of uncomplicated diabetes.

[91] Texon M The causes of heart disease a critique Bull N Y Acad Med. Oct 1989; 65(8): 836–841.

[92] The Great Cholesterol Con Anthony Colpo (Lulu) and The Great Cholesterol Con Dr Malcolm Kendrick (John Blake)

[93] Dr Richard Bernstein, "Diabetes Solution: the complete guide to achieving normal blood sugars"

[94] www.fpa.org.uk/

[95] AACE/ACE Guidelines CLINICAL PRACTICE GUIDELINES FOR HEALTHY EATING FOR THE PREVENTION AND TREATMENT OF METABOLIC AND ENDOCRINE DISEASES IN ADULTS:ENDOCRINE PRACTICE Vol 19 (Suppl 3) September/October 2013 1

[96] Dr Bernstein's Diabetes Solution Dr Richard Bernstein Brown and Little

[97] This amount of protein is judged on the weight of the total food – so 1oz/285g of chicken, eggs, fish and meat would make up the protein total, rather than the actual protein content of the food.

[98] Exposing the hidden dangers of iron. Ed Weinberg PhD Cumberland House

[99] Association of Dietary, Circulating, and Supplement Fatty Acids With Coronary Risk: A Systematic Review and Meta-analysis, Annals of Internal Medicine, published March 18

[100] Point: Postprandial Glucose Levels Are a Clinically Important Treatment TargetAntonio Ceriello, MD http://www.ncbi.nlm.nih.gov/pmc/articles/PMC2909084/

[101] Exposing the Hidden Dangers of Iron E.D. Weinberg PhD Cumberland House

[102] Dr Bernstein's Diabetes Solution Dr Richard K Bernstein Brown and Little

[103] One well-known salad dressing brand contains, for example, corn syrup, high fructose corn syrup, soybean oil, potassium sorbate, calcium disodium and disodium guanylate. Nice.

[104] Fats that Heal, Fats that Kill Udo Erasmus

[105] Yam D, Eliraz A, Berry EM Department of Membrane Research and Biophysics, Weizmann Institute of Science, Rehovot, Israel. Israel Journal of Medical Sciences [1996, 32(11):1134-1143] Diet and disease- -the Israeli paradox: possible dangers of a high omega-6 polyunsaturated fatty acid diet.

[106] Know your fats Mary Enig

[107] DIETARY CONJUGATED LINOLEIC ACID IN HEALTH: Physiological Effects and Mechanisms of Action1 Annual Review of Nutrition Vol. 22: 505-531 July 2002 Martha A. Belury

[108] Fats that Heal, Fats that Kill Udo Erasmus

[109] "Induction flu" when starting a low-carbohydrate diet is common as people's bodies adjust from burning glucose to burning fat for energy. Symptoms can include headaches, nausea and a lack of energy and they can last for a few days. To help yourself, drink lots and lots of water or herbal tea, and take a multi-mineral/multi-vitamin, as well as adding salt to your meals.

[110] Turmeric is known for its anti-inflammatory properties, whilst cinnamon and black pepper, thanks to its chromium content, are thought to provide blood-sugar lowering effects for people with type 2 diabetes.

[111] Too Much Sitting: The Population-Health Science of Sedentary Behaviour - http://www.ncbi.nlm.nih.gov/pmc/articles/PMC3404815/

[112] http://www.sciencedaily.com/releases/2010/03/100311123639.htm

[113] The World Health Organisation: http://www.who.int/mediacentre/factsheets/fs312/en/

Printed in Great Britain
by Amazon